Keto CrockPot Cookbook

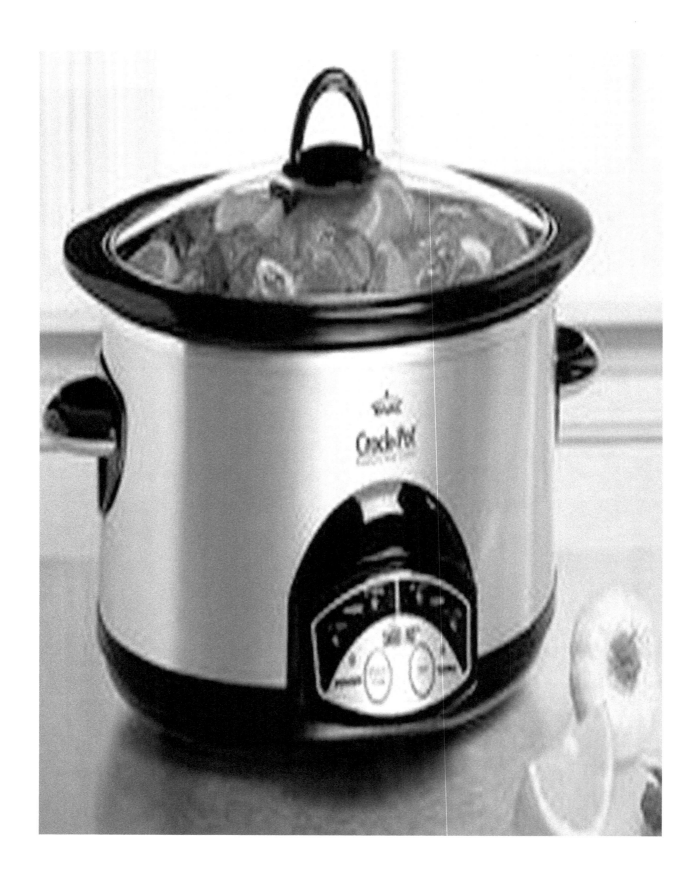

Keto CrockPot Cookbook

Healthy and Easy Ketogenic CrockPot Recipes for Lose Weight Forever and Live Better (Low carb crock-pot for weight loss)

Elena Jennifer

TABLE OF CONTENTS

Introduction

You might have heard of a Keto Diet Plan, but may not have an exact idea about what it exactly is or you might be hearing it for the very first time.

Whatever category you fall into, doesn't worry, I'm here to help you. As you landed up here, it means that you have some serious interest in knowing about diet and would like to get a handy list of easy Keto Crock Pot recipes for fat loss. It's quite evident that the well-known advice to "eat less and exercise more" for weight loss is not working for all of us. It is a fact that a significant portion of dieters who lose weight, gain it back quickly. So the real question is, is there an ultimate solution to this universal problem? As per my experience and research in this area, I have come up to a conclusion that keto diet is something which can help solve this problem of weight loss.

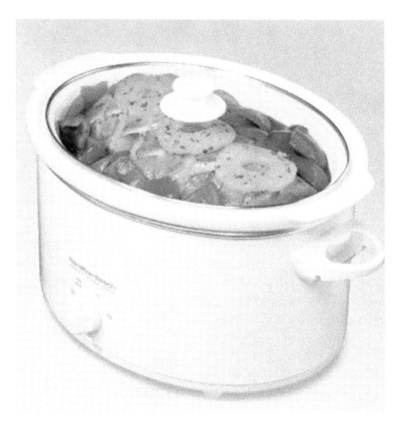

Ketosis is significant for your weight loss as it helps suppress your appetite unlike other diets and it also provides mental clarity and increases focus. Moreover, for preparing Keto Meals, crock pots are using, which will increase the nutritional benefits like anything. Once you get on track with Keto Diet, you no longer have to worry about your appetite. No more counting calories and no more crazy spot exercises to reduce your belly.

If this idea seems appealing to you, continue reading and get ready to be on a Keto Diet with delicious and healthy Crock Pot prepared meal plans. However, if you still have some questions, we will cover the entire upcoming chapter so that you can get started.

What is a Crock Pot?

Well, this can be a tricky question. Many people use the term "Crock Pot" to refer to a slow cooker, regardless of the brand or make. In fact, there is an official "Crock Pot", which is the slow cooker we will be using and referring to in this book.

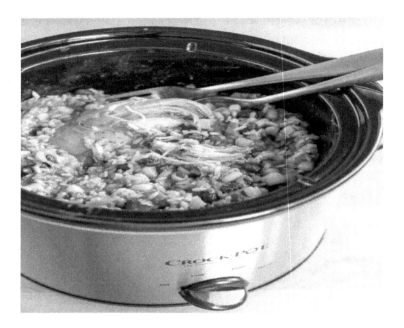

When talking about slow cookers in general, I would describe them as a "One-Pot" appliance which allows the user to cook dishes slowly and without need for supervision. The Crock Pot is most commonly known for slow-cooked meat dishes, stews, and soups, due to the long cook time and even heat distribution.

What is the Ketogenic Diet?

Unlike many other diets, this one is easy to understand! The Ketogenic Diet is simply a high fat, low carbohydrate diet that involves reducing your intake of carbs and replacing them with fats. When you eat foods that are high in carbs, your body produces two things: insulin and glucose.

1. Glucose is a molecule needed by our bodies to convert and use the energy from the food we eat to fuel our body, typically carbohydrate.
2. Insulin is a substance made by our pancreas to process glucose within our bloodstream.

Since glucose is our main source of energy, the fat we have stored away is therefore not needed and sits there unused. When deciding if the Ketogenic diet is for them, many people choose a typical diet of eating foods high in carbs. We have been taught that carbs are needed for energy since we were tots. This is true, but only to point.

Despite what you may have read, there are four types of Ketogenic diet.

1. High-protein Ketogenic Diet:

This type of keto diet involves eating lots of protein. The ratio required to stick to this type of diet is 60% fat, 35% protein and 5% carbohydrates.

2. Targeted Ketogenic Diet (TKD):

If you like the freedom of having some room to move around on diet, this one is for you! You can intake more carbs if you are working out as well.

3. Cyclical Ketogenic Diet (CKD):

This type requires periods of high-carb intake-for example, 5 Ketogenic days paired with a few high-carb consumption days.

4. Standard Ketogenic Diet (SKD):

This type of keto diet is the most popular and recommended. It requires you to consume moderate amounts of protein and high amounts of fat. It is based around this popular macro; 75% fat, 20% protein and 5% carbs.

The standard Ketogenic diet is the most popular diet for beginners, but you may find that the other three diets are better suited to your body and personal goals. For now, however, I suggest that you start with the standard Ketogenic diet to see how your body adapts and to minimize any side affects you may experience on the diet. Many of my students also start with the standard diet and their weight loss results have been excellent because they have exceeded my expectations every time.

Useful Tips and Tricks for Successful Keto Diet:

Here are some hacks on how to flourish with your Ketogenic diet:

1. Super-hydrate yourself by drinking 140 to 180 oz. of water each day.
2. Exercise regularly to activate GLUT-4, a molecule that pulls sugar from the bloodstream to store as glycogen I the muscles and liver.
3. Eat fermented foods to induce good bowel motility. Constipation may hinder ketosis.
4. Create more peace and relaxation in life because chronic stress lessens the ability to maintain ketosis.

5. Get enough sleep to preserve hormones and good blood circulation.
6. Increase salt intake to 3-5 grams daily. Himalayan pink salt comes handy.
7. Use medium-chain triglyceride oil regularly as they are readily metabolized to ketone bodies.
8. Taking ketone supplements are beneficial especially at the onset of your Ketogenic journey.
9. Never exceed 20 or 30 grams of carbohydrates daily. Always count your carbs. Remember this formula: Total carbs-Fiber = Net carbs.

Be wary of eating out. Never be shy to ask for alternatives and customized meals to suit your Ketogenic diet.

How to Use the Crock Pot?

The Crock Pot is incredibly easy to use! That's part of the major appeal of this genius appliance. There are not many ways you can mess up your food with the Crock Pots, but there are some tips to follow to ensure a successful result!

1. Temperature:

Most Crock Pot models have a LOW and HIGH setting. You need to adjust your cooking time according to the temperature setting. For example, if you have the HIGH setting on, your dish might take 4 hours to cook, but if you have the LOW setting on, it might take 8 hours. Follow the guidelines in your Crock Pot handbook, and stick to the time suggestions in these recipes (and others!).

2. Size and Servings:

When purchasing your Crock Pot, choose a size that suits your regular serving needs; i.e. if you have a family of 5, choose a large pot. The thing is, you should never over-fill the Crock Pot. If you add too many ingredients, the food won't cook evenly, and it might turn out sloppy and flavorless. Don't fill the Crock Pot more than two thirds full and you'll be fine!

3. Time:

If you'd like to cook your meal throughout the day, while you are out and about, you can do so! Choose a LOW setting and cook the meal slowly, for at least 8 hours (or according to the recipe instructions). When the meal has finished cooking, the Crock Pot will automatically switch to WARM until you are ready to devour your meal.

4. Liquids:

Crock Pots and slow cookers do not reduce liquids. When you are cooking in a regular pot or pan, the liquid you add will evaporate, thicken, and reduce: this does not happen when cooking with the Crock Pot! The liquid you add at the start will be there at the end. Therefore, be careful with the amount of liquid you are adding to your dish. You can reduce and simmer liquids such as wine and cream in a pot or fry pan before you add it to the slow cooker. When using a recipe made especially for a Crock Pot or Slow Cooker, follow it carefully and you'll be perfectly fine.

What are the Benefits of Using the Crock Pot?

Anyone who owns and uses a Crock Pot will have to you about the many benefits of this appliance! Here are some of the fantastic reasons to incorporate the Crock Pot into your cooking routine:

1. Convenience:

Instead of hauling out an armful of pots and pans from the cupboards, just use the Crock Pot! It's already there on the bench, so load it up. All you need to do is clean the inner pot after you're done, and put it back into the Crock Pot unit, ready for next time.

2. Ready-to-go Meals:

A crazy lifestyle doesn't mean that you need to sacrifice wholesome and delicious meals. The amazing thing about the Crock Pot is that you can leave it to cook your meal while you are at work, or even overnight. Load the ingredients into the pot, set the temperature and time, and walk away.

3. Tender Meat:

Slow cooked meat is tender, melt-in-the-mouth, and satisfying. You can achieve this by simply throwing the meat into the pot with any flavorings you like, a small amount of liquid, and simply forget about it for hours while you live your life!

4. Versatility:

As you will see in the recipe section, you can cook anything in the Crock Pot! Meat, Vegetables, Seafood, Dessert, Starters! You can cook your dish entirely in the Crock Pot, from start to finish, or you can finish it off in a hot fry pan to give a golden crunch to meat and veggie dishes.

What to Avoid?

The Ketogenic Diet discourages the consumption of carbohydrate that is converted to glucose. Thus said, dieters are discouraged to eat high amounts of sugar and starch. These include rice, potatoes, bread, pasta, and other sugary beverages. But more than sugary foods and starches, what are other types of foods that you need to avoid when following the Ketogenic diet.

1. Sugary Foods:

Sugary foods such as cakes, candies, and ice cream should be avoided. But aside from these sinful foods, even foods that are marketed as health products are discouraged under the Ketogenic diet. These include fruit juices and sodas.

2. Root Vegetables:

Root vegetables contain high amounts of starch and must, therefore be avoided. These include carrots, parsnips, potatoes, and other types of tubers.

3. Fruits:

As mentioned earlier, fruits are discouraged under the Ketogenic diet. But if you are craving for fruits, you are limited to consuming berries like strawberries, cherries, and many others.

4. Beans:

Beans such as white beans, red beans, lentils, pulses, and basically all types of beans are discouraged with the Ketogenic diet.

5. Low Carb Products:

Many low-carb products are marketed and touted for their health benefits but not on the Ketogenic diet. You need to increase the amount of fat that you can get and dairy products, for example, are good sources. So instead of opting for low-fat milk, opt for the full-fat version.

6. Alcohol:

Specifically, beer contains high amounts of carbohydrates but distilled drinks and wine can be consumed under limited amounts.

Chicken Recipes

Comforting Chicken Stew:

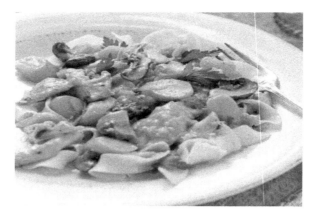

Serves: 6
Preparation Time: 20 minutes
Cooking Time: 6 hours
Macros per serving:
Calories: 203
Protein: 26.9 grams
Fat: 6.8 grams
Carbohydrates: 7 grams

What you'll need:

- 3 cups carrots, peeled and cubed
- ½ cup yellow onion, chopped
- 2 garlic cloves, minced
- Salt and freshly ground black pepper, to taste
- ¼ teaspoon dried thyme
- ½ teaspoon dried sage
- 3 (6-ounce) grass-fed, boneless chicken breasts, cubed
- 2 cups homemade chicken broth

How to make it:

1. In a large Crockpot, add all ingredients except cilantro and stir to combine.
2. Set the Crockpot on low and cook, covered, for about 7-8 hours
3. Serve hot.

Crock Pot Balsamic Boneless Chicken Thighs:

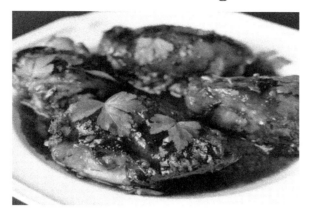

Serves: 8
Preparation Time: 5 minutes
Cooking Time: 4 hours
Macros per serving:
Calories: 133
Protein: 20.1 grams
Fat: 4 grams
Carbohydrates: 5.6 grams

What you'll need:

- 1 teaspoon Ground garlic
- 1 teaspoon Basil dried
- ½ teaspoon Salt
- ½ teaspoon Pepper
- 2 teaspoons Onion, dried & minced
- 4 Minced garlic cloves
- 1 tablespoon Olive oil, extra virgin
- ½ cup Balsamic vinegar
- 8 Chicken thighs boneless and skinless (about 24 ounces)
- Fresh chopped parsley

How to make it:

1. Take a medium bowl and mix the all dry spices and paste all over the chicken.
2. Pour one tablespoon olive oil to the Crockpot.
3. Add garlic.
4. Place the chicken.
5. You can dispense the balsamic vinegar on the chicken and make sure it reaches everywhere on the chicken.
6. Cover the crockpot and cook on high about 4 hours.
7. Once cooking over, transfer the dish to a serving bowl.
8. Sprinkle fresh on top the chicken.
9. Serve and enjoy.

Chicken Tikka Masala:

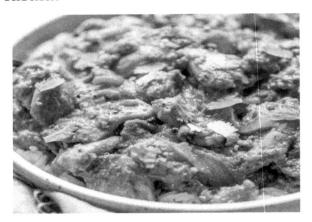

Serves: 2
Preparation Time: 15 minutes
Cooking Time: 6 hours
Macros per serving:
Calories: 493
Protein: 46 grams
Fat: 41.2 grams
Carbohydrates: 5.8 grams

What you'll need:

- 1 lb. chicken thighs, de-boned and chopped into bite-sized
- 3 teaspoons gram masala
- ½ cup heavy cream
- ½ cup coconut milk
- 1 teaspoon onion powder
- 2 minced cloves of garlic
- 1 teaspoon paprika
- 2 teaspoons salt

How to make it:

1. Put chicken to Crockpot and add grated ginger knob on top. Also add the seasonings: 1 teaspoon onion powder, 2 minced cloves of garlic, 1 teaspoon paprika and 2 teaspoons salt. Mix.
2. Add tomatoes and coconut oil. Mix.
3. Cook for 6 hours on low.
4. When cooked, add heavy cream to chicken the curry.

Flavorful Chicken and Gravy:

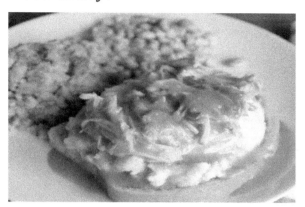

Serves: 6

Preparation Time: 10 minutes

Cooking Time: 8 hours

Macros per serving:

Calories: 323

Protein: 44.9 grams

Fat: 12 grams

Carbohydrates: 6.2 grams

What you'll need:

- 2 lbs. chicken breasts, skinless, boneless and cut into pieces
- 3 cups chicken stock
- 1 oz. brown gravy mix
- 1 oz. onion soup mix

How to make it:

1. Add chicken stock, brown gravy mix, and onion soup mix into the slow cooker and stir well.
2. Add chicken into the slow cooker.
3. Cover and cook on low for 8 hours.
4. Stir well and serve.

Lemon Grass and Coconut Chicken:

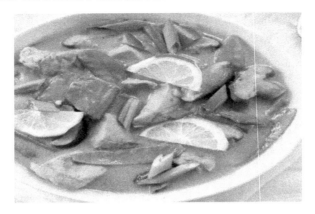

Serves: 6
Preparation Time: 20 minutes
Cooking Time: 5 hours
Macros per serving:
Calories: 455
Protein: 40.89 grams
Fat: 29.57 grams
Carbohydrates: 5.38 grams

What you'll need:

- 10 chicken drumsticks, skin removed
- Salt and pepper to taste
- 1 stalk of lemongrass, trimmed
- 4 cloves of garlic, minced
- 1 pieces ginger, sliced thinly
- 1 cup coconut milk
- 3 tablespoons coconut aminos
- 2 tablespoons fish sauce
- 1 teaspoon five spice powder
- 1 green onion, chopped

How to make it:

1. In a large bowl, season the chicken drumstick with salt and pepper.
2. Place the lemongrass, garlic, ginger, coconut milk, coconut aminos, fish sauce, and five-spice powder in a blender or food processor. Blend until smooth.
3. Place the chicken in the slow cooker and pour over the marinade. Mix well.
4. Set the Crockpot to low and cook for 4 to 5 hours.
5. Once done, serve with green onions.

Indian Chicken Curry:

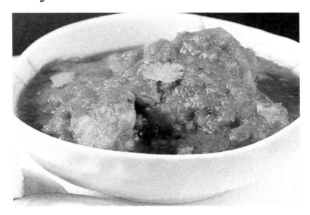

Serves: 6
Preparation Time: 20 minutes
Cooking Time: 5 hours 5 minutes
Macros per serving:
Calories: 426
Protein: 50.8 grams
Fat: 17.5 grams
Carbohydrates: 11.6 grams

What you'll need:

- 2 pounds grass-fed, bone-in chicken thighs
- Salt and freshly ground black pepper, to taste
- 1 small yellow onion, chopped roughly
- 3 garlic cloves, chopped roughly
- 1 teaspoon fresh ginger, chopped roughly
- 1 tablespoon curry powder
- ¼ cup water
- 2 tablespoons olive oil
- 1 cup cherry tomatoes, halved
- 1 ¼ cups plain yogurt, whipped
- ¼ cup fresh cilantro
- 1 tablespoon fresh lemon juice

How to make it:

1. Season chicken thighs with salt and black pepper evenly.
2. In a food processor, add onion, garlic, ginger, water, and curry powder and pulse until smooth.
3. In a frying pan, heat oil and sauté onion mixture for about 3-5 minutes.
4. In a large Crockpot, place chicken thighs with sautéed onion mixture, tomatoes, and yogurt and stir to combine.
5. Set the Crockpot on low and cook, covered, for about 5 hours.
6. Stir in cilantro and lemon juice and serve hot.

Crock Pot Chicken Lo Mein:

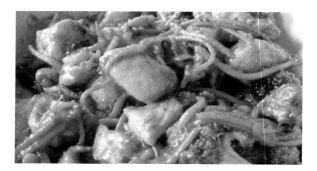

Serves: 6
Preparation Time: 10 minutes
Cooking Time: 4 hours
Macros per serving:
Calories: 174
Protein: 24.5 grams
Fat: 10.2 grams
Carbohydrates: 3.1 grams
What you'll need:

- 1 ½ pounds Chicken sliced
- 1 bunch Napa cabbage washed
- 12 ounces Low carb noodles
- 1 teaspoon Clove garlic, minced
- Salt to taste
- Pepper as required

For Marinating:

- 1 tablespoon Tamari/soy aminos
- ½ teaspoon Garlic paste
- ½ teaspoon Sesame oil

For making sauce:

- ¾ cup Chicken broth
- 1 tablespoon Sweetener
- ¼ cup Tamari/soy aminos
- 1 tablespoon Vinegar
- 2 teaspoons Sesame oil
- 1 teaspoon Pepper chili flakes
- ½ teaspoon Thickener (optional)

How to make it:

1. Marinate the chicken using the ingredients and keep it in the fridge for setting about 30 minutes. Use a small bowl to marinate.
2. Clean the Crockpot and coat slightly with non-stick oil.
3. Put the marinated chicken in the cooker and start cooking in slow heat for about 2 hours.
4. Stir it intermittently and also check the tenderness of the chicken.
5. Once done, remove the chicken from the cooker and put garlic, ginger, and vegetables into the cooker and place the cooked chicken on top of it.
6. Now it is time for making the sauce.
7. Mix all the sauce ingredients in a bowl and transfer everything to the cooker.
8. Continue cook for about 2 hours and stir intermittently.
9. Ten minutes before winding up the cooking, rinse the noodle and keep it ready.
10. Transfer the washed and soaked noodles into the cooker.
11. Cover the noodles with the sauce by using tongs.
12. Add the thickener if required.
13. Just pot the Crockpot to a high temperature for about 15 minutes.
14. Serve hot

Roasted Chicken with Lemon & Parsley Butter:

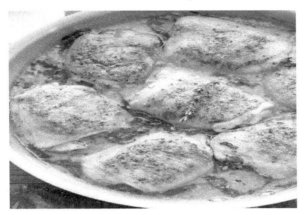

Serves: 2
Preparation Time: 5 minutes
Cooking Time: 8 hours
Macros per serving:
Calories: 300
Protein: 29 grams
Fat: 18 grams
Carbohydrates: 1 gram

What you'll need:

- 4 lb. chicken, any part
- 1 whole lemon, sliced
- 2 tablespoons butter or ghee
- 1 tablespoon parsley, chopped

How to make it:

1. Rub chicken all over with salt and pepper to taste. Put in the Crockpot and pour 1 cup of water.
2. Cover and cook for 3 hours on high.
3. When cooked, add the lemon slices butter and parsley to the Crockpot.
4. Cook and cover for another 10 minutes.

Tender Cilantro Lime Chicken:

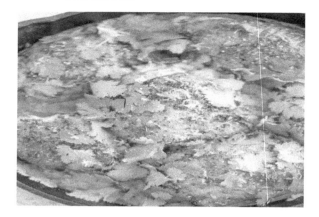

Serves: 12
Preparation Time: 10 minutes
Cooking Time: 6 hours
Macros per serving:
Calories: 162
Protein: 22.4 grams
Fat: 5.9 grams
Carbohydrates: 4.5 grams

What you'll need:

- 6 chicken breast, boneless
- 2 jalapeno peppers, chopped
- 1.25 oz. taco seasoning
- ¼ cup fresh cilantro, chopped
- 1 lime juice
- 24 oz. salsa

How to make it:

1. Add all ingredients except chicken into the slow cooker and mix well.
2. Add chicken into the slow cooker.
3. Cover and cook on low for 6 hours.
4. Shred chicken using a fork and serve.

Keto Jerk Chicken:

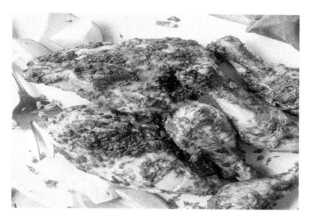

Serves: 4
Preparation Time: 10 minutes
Cooking Time: 5 hours
Macros per serving:
Calories: 281
Protein: 30.24 grams
Fat: 15.38 grams
Carbohydrates: 4.31 grams

What you'll need:

- 4 teaspoons paprika
- 4 teaspoons salt
- 1 teaspoon cayenne pepper
- 2 teaspoons thyme
- 2 teaspoons onion powder
- 2 teaspoons garlic powder
- 1 teaspoon black pepper
- 5 chicken drumsticks, skin removed

How to make it:

1. Make a spice rub by combining in bowl paprika, salt, cayenne pepper, thyme, onion powder, garlic powder, and black pepper.
2. Coat the chicken with the spice rub and place inside the Crockpot.
3. Set the temperature to low heat and cook for 6 hours or until the chicken meat falls off the bone.

Sweet and Tangy Chicken:

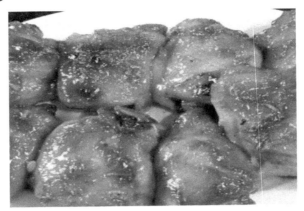

Serves: 6
Preparation Time: 15 minutes
Cooking Time: 8 hours
Macros per serving:
Calories: 254
Protein: 37.4 grams
Fat: 9.6 grams
Carbohydrates: 6 grams

What you'll need:

- 1 medium yellow onion, chopped
- 1/3 cup chives, minced
- 1 tablespoon fresh ginger, minced
- 3 tablespoons fresh lemon juice
- 2 tablespoons erythritol
- 2 tablespoons water
- 1 ½ tablespoons soy sauce
- ½ teaspoon red pepper flakes
- 2 ½ pounds grass-fed boneless chicken breasts, cut into pieces

How to make it:

1. In a bowl, add all ingredients except chicken and blend well.
2. Place chicken pieces in the bottom of a Crockpot and top evenly with onion mixture.
3. Set the Crockpot on low and cook, covered for about 6-8 hours.
4. Serve hot

Slow Cooker Moscow Chicken:

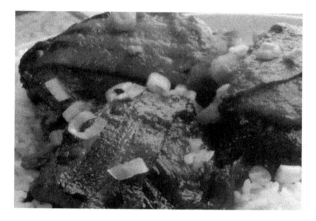

Serves: 6
Preparation Time: 10-15 minutes
Cooking Time: 6 hours
Macros per serving:
Calories: 150.7
Protein: 14.9 grams
Fat: 2.8 grams
Carbohydrates: 10.8 grams

What you'll need:

- 6 Chicken thighs
- ½ teaspoon Grated ginger
- 6 Bacon, sliced
- 10 ounces Russian salad dressing
- 2 Clove garlic, chopped
- 2 Onion, chopped
- Pepper as required
- Salt to taste

How to make it:

1. Take a large skillet and heat on medium temperature.
2. Put chicken and cook it until both sides become brown.
3. Let it cool after done.
4. Now warp the chicken thighs in bacon and put it into the slow cooker.
5. Spread ginger and garlic over the chicken.
6. Top it with Russian salad.
7. Cook for 5-6 hours
8. Once ready, season it with pepper and salt.

Greek Chicken:

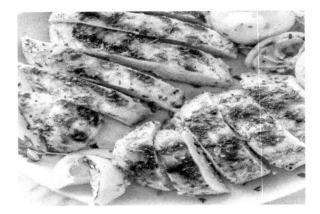

Serves: 2
Preparation Time: 5 minutes
Cooking Time: 6 hours
Macros per serving:
Calories: 396
Protein: 28.7 grams
Fat: 29.8 grams
Carbohydrates: 4 grams

What you'll need:

- 2 chicken breast, skinless
- 1 ½ tablespoon Greek Rub
- 1 ½ tablespoons lemon juice
- 1 chicken bouillon cube dissolved in water

How to make it:

1. Coat each breast with Greek rub, and then rub with garlic powder.
2. Put the chicken breasts in the Crockpot and spray with lemon juice.
3. Pour the chicken bouillon mixture in the Crockpot.
4. Cook for 6 hours on low.

Delicious Butter Chicken:

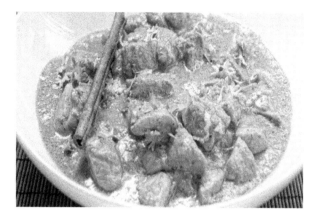

Serves: 8
Preparation Time: 10 minutes
Cooking Time: 6 hours 30 minutes
Macros per serving:
Calories: 374
Protein: 37.5 grams
Fat: 22.5 grams
Carbohydrates: 5.3 grams

What you'll need:

- 2.2 lbs. chicken thighs, skinless
- 1 cup coconut milk
- 1 cup tomatoes, crushed
- 4 tablespoons butter
- 2 teaspoons curry powder
- 2 teaspoons ground cumin
- 2 teaspoons ground paprika
- 3 teaspoons ground cinnamon
- 1 medium onion, chopped
- 1 teaspoon salt

How to make it:

1. Add onion into the slow cooker then place chicken on top of onion.
2. Sprinkle all spices on top of chicken.
3. Pour crushed tomatoes on top of chicken.
4. Cover and cook on low for 6 hours.
5. Add coconut milk and cook for one more half-hour.
6. Stir well and serve.

Easy-Breezy Fajita Chicken:

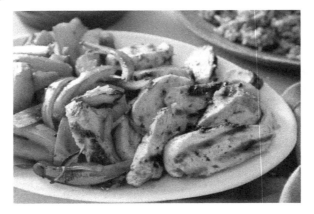

Serves: 8
Preparation Time: 10 minutes
Cooking Time: 6 hours
Macros per serving:
Calories: 151
Protein: 26.18 grams
Fat: 3.13 grams
Carbohydrates: 3.44 grams

What you'll need:

- 2 pounds boneless chicken breast, skin removed
- 1 small onion, sliced thinly
- 4 cloves of garlic, minced
- 2 cups bell pepper, sliced
- 1 can diced tomatoes
- 1 teaspoon salt
- 1 teaspoon oregano
- 1 teaspoon coriander, ground
- ½ teaspoon cumin
- ½ teaspoon chili powder

How to make it:

1. Place the chicken at the bottom of the Crockpot and add the onions, garlic and bell peppers.
2. Pour over the diced tomatoes.
3. Stir in the rest of the ingredients.
4. Cook at the low-temperature setting for 6 hours.

Beef Recipes

Soul Warming Beef Stew:

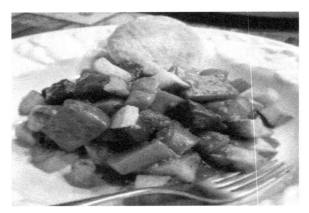

Serves: 8
Preparation Time: 15 minutes
Cooking Time: 9 hours
Macros per serving:
Calories: 248
Protein: 36.5 grams
Fat: 7.4 grams
Carbohydrates: 7.4 grams

What you'll need:

- 1 medium head cabbage, roughly chopped (485 g)
- 1 medium yellow onion, chopped
- 6 garlic cloves, minced
- 2 pounds grass-fed beef stew meat, cubed
- 2 cups tomatoes, chopped finely
- Salt and freshly ground black pepper, to taste
- 1 cup homemade beef broth

How to make it:

1. In a large Crockpot, add all ingredients and stir to combine.
2. Set the Crockpot on low and cook, covered, for about 9 hours.
3. Serve hot.

Crockpot – Low Carb Short Beef Ribs:

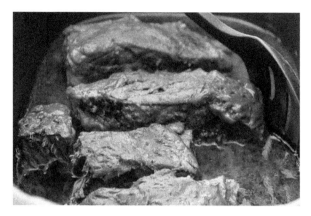

Serves: 12
Preparation Time: 15 minutes
Cooking Time: 4 hours
Macros per serving:
Calories: 489
Protein: 16 grams
Fat: 42 grams
Carbohydrates: 3 grams

What you'll need:

- 4 pounds Beef with short ribs or boneless
- 1 ½ cups Onion, chopped
- 1 cup Beef broth
- 2 tablespoons Olive oil
- 2 tablespoons Worcestershire sauce or ordinary homemade
- 2 tablespoons Tomato paste
- 3 No's Garlic clove, minced
- Salt to taste
- Pepper to taste
- 1 ½ cups Red wine
- Celery, carrots – optional

How to make it:

1. In a large skillet, pour oil and heat on medium temperature.
2. Season the ribs, one side with salt and pepper.
3. Put half of the ribs, facing the seasoned into the hot oil.
4. Flip it once the side becomes brown.
5. Remove and set aside.
6. Continue the remaining.
7. Take a 4-quart Crockpot and place short ribs into it.
8. In the skillet put the remaining ingredients and boil it.
9. Cook until the onion becomes tender.
10. Transfer it to the Crockpot.
11. Cover and continue cooking for 8-10 hours.

Braised Corned beef Brisket:

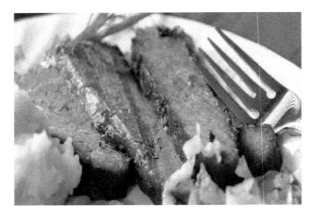

Serves: 2
Preparation Time: 15 minutes
Cooking Time: 6 hours 15 minutes
Macros per serving:
Calories: 455
Protein: 30.6 grams
Fat: 33.7 grams
Carbohydrates: 5.4 grams

What you'll need:

- 1/3 tablespoon vegetable oil
- 1/3 flat-cut corned beef brisket
- 1/3 tablespoon browning sauce

How to make it:

1. Prepare seasonings: 1/3 sliced onion and 2 sliced garlic cloves.
2. Apply a generous amount of browning sauce to both sides of the brisket.
3. In a skillet, cook the brisket in preheated vegetable oil for 5-8 minutes on both sides.
4. Place the brisket in a crock-pot. Scatter the seasonings and add a tablespoon of water.
5. Cover and cook for 6 hours on low.

Chili Lime Shredded Beef:

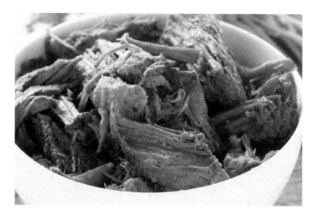

Serves: 6
Preparation Time: 10 minutes
Cooking Time: 8 hours
Macros per serving:

Calories: 563
Protein: 40.2 grams
Fat: 42.5 grams
Carbohydrates: 2.5 grams

What you'll need:

- 2 lb. beef chuck roast
- 2 lime juice
- 3 garlic cloves, crushed
- 1 teaspoon chili powder
- 4 cups chicken stock
- 1 teaspoon salt

How to make it:

1. Place chuck roast into the bottom of slow cooker.
2. Pour chicken stock over chuck roast
3. Season roast with chili powder, garlic, and salt.
4. Cover and cook on low for 8 hours.
5. Shred chuck roast using a fork and pour lime juice over shredded meat.
6. Serve hot and enjoy.

Exotic Middle Eastern Beef:

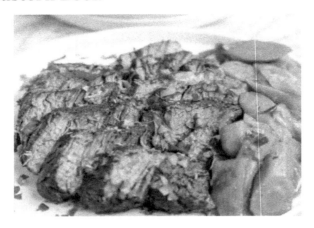

Serves: 8
Preparation Time: 20 minutes
Cooking Time: 8 hours
Macros per serving:
Calories: 563
Protein: 40.91 grams
Fat: 40.86 grams
Carbohydrates: 5.14 grams

What you'll need:

- 3 pounds beef brisket
- Salt and pepper to taste
- 1 teaspoon fennel seeds
- 1 teaspoon whole peppercorns
- 1 teaspoon cumin powder
- 1 teaspoon cardamom powder
- ½ teaspoon ground cinnamon
- 3 tablespoons tomato paste
- ½ onion, chopped
- 3 cups bone broth
- ¼ cup coconut vinegar

How to make it:

1. Place all ingredients in the pot.
2. Cook at low temperature for 8 hours.
3. Once cooked, shred with a fork.

Richly Taste Beef Chili:

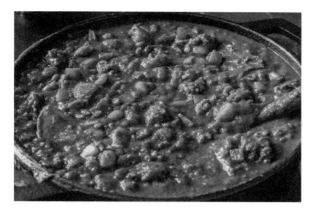

Serves: 12
Preparation Time: 20 minutes
Cooking Time: 7 hours
Macros per serving:
Calories: 303
Protein: 41.2 grams
Fat: 10.7 grams
Carbohydrates: 10.9 grams

What you'll need:

- 3 pounds ground lean grass-fed beef
- 1 large yellow onion, chopped
- Salt and freshly ground black pepper, to taste
- 1 (10-ounces) package Portobello mushrooms, sliced
- 1 (28-ounce) can fire-roasted tomatoes with juice
- 2 jalapeno peppers, seeded and chopped finely
- 1 tablespoon garlic, minced
- 3 tablespoons capers
- ¼ cup sugar-free tomato paste
- 1 cup homemade beef broth
- 2 tablespoons dried thyme, crushed
- 2 tablespoons ground cumin
- 1 tablespoon ground cinnamon
- 3 tablespoons red chili powder
- 1 tablespoon cayenne pepper
- ½ tablespoon erythritol
- 2 tablespoons balsamic vinegar
- 1 ¼ cups parmesan cheese, grated freshly
- 2 cups scallions, chopped

How to make it:

1. In a large Crockpot, add beef, onion, salt, and black pepper and stir well.
2. Set the Crockpot on low and cook, covered, for about 3 hours, stirring occasionally.
3. Uncover the Crockpot and drain the grease completely.
4. Add remaining ingredients except for parmesan cheese and scallion and mix well.
5. Set the Crockpot on low and cook, covered, for about 3-4 hours
6. Serve hot with the topping of cheese and scallion.

Mexican Crockpot Beef Roast:

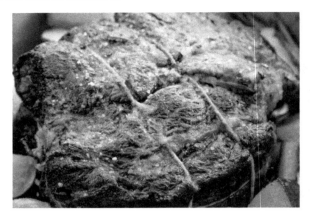

Serves: 10
Preparation Time: 15 minutes
Cooking Time: 7 hours
Macros per serving:
Calories: 608
Protein: 44 grams
Fat: 3 grams
Carbohydrates: 7 grams

What you'll need:

- 3 ½ pounds Beef chuck arm
- 1 teaspoon Cumin, grounded
- 2 teaspoons Garlic, minced
- 1 teaspoon Black pepper, ground
- 2 tablespoons Tomato paste
- ½ teaspoon Coriander, grounded
- 2 cups Fresh salsa
- 3 tablespoons Bacon grease
- 2 cups Beef broth
- 2 tablespoons Sauce
- Salt to taste

How to make it:

1. Season the beef with grounded black pepper and spices.
2. Take a heavy skillet and over medium-high heat, melt the bacon grease.
3. Roast it until becoming brown on all sides.
4. Put all the roasted beef in the crockpot.
5. Add tomato paste, sauce and salsa over the meet.
6. Add beef broth.
7. Put the remaining bacon grease and any other leftovers over the beef.
8. Cover the cook on low heat.
9. Depending on the meet, you need to cook it for 6-8 hours on slow cooking.
10. Once the cooking is over, remove the beef to a large bowl and pull the meat into small rags, when it is cool. You can do it by hand or with forks. Remove excess fat if anything is there.
11. Once done, serve hot.

Italian Beef for Sandwiches:

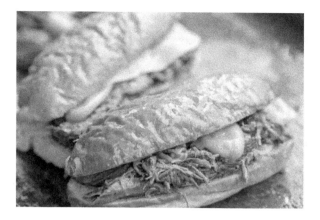

Serves: 2
Preparation Time: 15 minutes
Cooking Time: 5 hours
Macros per serving:
Calories: 318
Protein: 39.4 grams
Fat: 15.8 grams
Carbohydrates: 1.6 grams

What you'll need:

- ¼ bay leaf
- ¼ (0.7 oz.) package dry Italian – style salad dressing mix
- ¼ teaspoon dried parsley
- ¼ teaspoon dried oregano
- ¼ (5 lb.) rump roast

How to make it:

1. Prepare to the season: ½ cup water with salt, garlic powder, and ground black pepper to taste.
2. Add the seasonings to the salad dressing mix.
3. Add the bay leaf, parsley, and oregano. Mix well.
4. Put the roast in the crock-pot and pour the resulting salad dressing mixture. Mix well.
5. Cover and cook for four to five hours on high.

Tasty Pulled Beef:

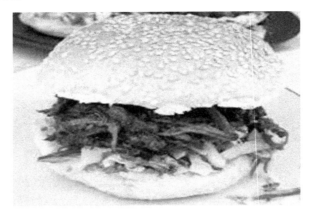

Serves: 12
Preparation Time: 10 minutes
Cooking Time: 8 hours 30 minutes
Macros per serving:
Calories: 582
Protein: 40.4 grams
Fat: 42.6 grams
Carbohydrates: 6.8 grams

What you'll need:

- 4 lbs. beef chuck roast
- 1 teaspoon onion powder
- 2 tablespoons chili powder
- 1 tablespoon paprika
- 2 garlic cloves, minced
- 1 tablespoon Dijon mustard
- 1 cup ketchup
- 1 cup balsamic vinegar
- 2 cups chicken stock
- Pepper
- Salt

How to make it:

1. In a bowl, combine together paprika. Garlic, onion powder, chili powder, pepper, and salt.
2. Rub spice mixture all over beef roasted and place in the slow cooker.
3. Pour chicken stock over roast. Cover slow cookware with lid and cook on low for eight hours.
4. Add ketchup, vinegar, mustard, pepper, and salt in a saucepan and heat over medium heat. Bring to boil and let simmer for ten minutes.
5. Remove beef roast from slow cooker and shred using a fork.
6. Return shredded meat into the slow cooker and pour ketchup mixture over shredded meat.
7. Stir well and cook on high for 30 minutes more.
8. Serve and enjoy.

Pepper Beef Tongue Stew:

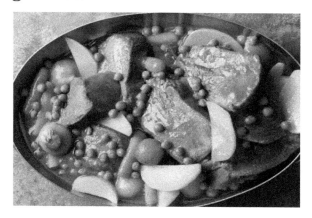

Serves: 10
Preparation Time: 15 minutes
Cooking Time: 8 hours
Macros per serving:
Calories: 441
Protein: 28.57 grams
Fat: 31.07 grams
Carbohydrates: 9.3 grams

What you'll need:

- 3 pounds sliced beef tongue, boiled and cleaned
- 1 Onion, chopped
- 6 cloves of garlic, minced
- 1 red bell pepper, diced
- 1 yellow bell pepper, diced
- 2 cups chicken stock
- 8-ounce can of tomato sauce
- 2 jalapeno peppers, diced
- Salt and pepper to taste
- 1 teaspoon Cajun spice
- 1 ¾ stick of butter
- 1 bunch of green onion, chopped

How to make it:

1. Place the beef tongue, onion, garlic, and bell peppers in the Crockpot.
2. Add the chicken stock and tomato sauce. Stir in the jalapeno pepper and season with salt, pepper and Cajun spice.
3. Cook on low temperature for 8 hours.
4. Once cooked, add butter and garnish with green onions.

Sweet & Tangy Beef Shoulder:

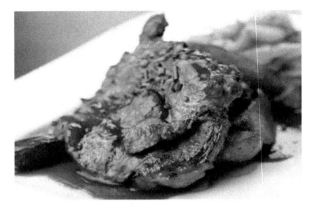

Serves: 14
Preparation Time: 15 minutes
Cooking Time: 9 hours 10 minutes
Macros per serving:
Calories: 516
Protein: 48.4 grams
Fat: 33.1 grams
Carbohydrates: 1.1 grams

What you'll need:

- ¼ cup unsalted butter
- 8 pounds grass-fed chuck shoulder roast
- Salt and freshly ground black pepper, to taste
- 1 yellow onion, chopped
- 4 garlic cloves, minced
- 1 tablespoon Dijon mustard
- 2 tablespoons vinegar
- 2 tablespoons fresh lemon juice
- 3-4 drops liquid stevia

How to make it:

1. In a large skillet, melt butter over medium-high heat and cook beef with salt and black pepper for about 1-2 minutes per side.
2. Transfer the beef into a large Crockpot.
3. In the same skillet, add onion and sauté for about 2-3 minutes.
4. Place onion evenly over beef.
5. In a bowl, mix together remaining ingredients.
6. Pour the sauce evenly over beef.
7. Set the Crockpot on low and cook, covered, for about 9 hours.
8. Uncover the Crockpot and transfer the beef to a cutting board.
9. Transfer the sauce into a small pan over medium-high heat and cook for about 5 minutes or until desired thickness.
10. Cut beef shoulder into desired sized slices.
11. Pour sauce over beef slices and serve.

Ronaldo's Beef Carnitas:

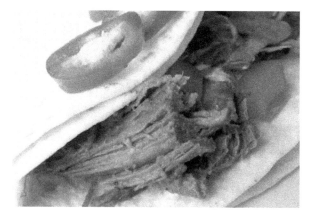

Serves: 2
Preparation Time: 5 minutes
Cooking Time: 8 hours
Macros per serving:
Calories: 218
Protein: 20.8 grams
Fat: 13.8 grams
Carbohydrates: 1.4 grams

What you'll need:

- 11 oz. chuck roast
- 1/8 can green chili peppers, chopped
- 1 teaspoon chili powder
- 1/8 teaspoon dried oregano
- 1/8 teaspoon ground cumin

How to make it:

1. Prepare the seasonings: mix all ingredients except the chuck roast. Add salt and pepper to taste.
2. Rub the mixture generously on the chuck roast and cover with aluminum foil. Put in the crock-pot.
3. Cover and cook for concerning eight hours on low.

Smokey Beef Brisket:

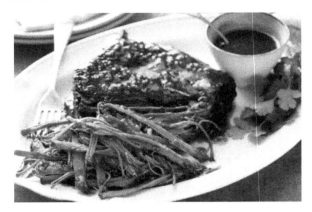

Serves: 6
Preparation Time: 10 minutes
Cooking Time 8 hours
Macros per serving:
Calories: 297
Protein: 46.5 grams
Fat: 9.8 grams
Carbohydrates: 2.2 grams

What you'll need:

- 2 lbs. beef brisket
- 3 tablespoons chili sauce
- ¼ cup chicken broth
- 1 ½ teaspoons liquid smoke
- ½ teaspoon pepper
- 1 teaspoon cumin
- 1 tablespoon Worcestershire sauce
- 1 tablespoon chili powder
- 3 garlic cloves, chopped
- ½ onion, chopped

How to make it:

1. In a small bowl, mix together chili powder, pepper, cumin, Worcestershire sauce, and garlic.
2. Rub chili powder mixture all over the beef brisket and place brisket into the slow cooker.
3. Mix together broth, chili sauce, onion, and liquid smoke and pour over brisket.
4. Cover and cook on low for 8 hours.
5. Remove brisket from slow cooker and slice and serve.

Indian Beef Stew:

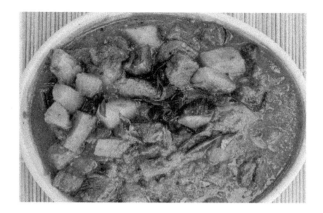

Serves: 8
Preparation Time: 20 minutes
Cooking Time: 8 hours
Macros per serving:
Calories: 134
Protein: 15.96 grams
Fat: 4.88 grams
Carbohydrates: 3.48 grams

What you'll need:

- ½ tablespoon oil
- 2 ½ pounds beef chunks
- 1 onion, diced
- 1 can tomatoes
- 2 cups beef stock
- 2 teaspoons ginger paste
- 2 teaspoons garlic, minced
- 2 tablespoons curry powder
- 2 teaspoons gram masala powder
- ¼ teaspoon ground cloves
- 2 bay leaves
- ¼ cup whipping cream
- ½ cup Greek yogurt

How to make it:

1. In a skillet, heat oil and sear the beef chunks. Set aside.
2. Place all ingredients in the Crockpot except the whipping cream and yogurt.
3. Add the seared beef chunks.
4. Close the lid and cook on low for eight hours.
5. Add the cream and yogurt before serving.

Divine Beef Shanks:

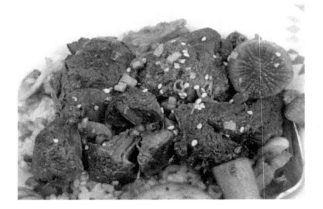

Serves: 10
Preparation Time: 15 minutes
Cooking Time: 8 hours 10 minutes
Macros per serving:
Calories: 513
Protein: 77.9 grams
Fat: 18.9 grams
Carbohydrates: 3.2 grams

What you'll need:

- 3 tablespoons unsalted butter
- 5 (1-pound) grass-fed beef shanks
- Salt and freshly ground black pepper, to taste
- 1 large yellow onion, chopped
- 10 garlic cloves, minced
- 2 tablespoons sugar-free tomato paste
- 4 fresh rosemary sprigs
- 4 fresh thyme sprigs
- 2 cups homemade beef broth

How to make it:

1. In a large skillet, melt butter over medium-high heat and cook beef shanks with salt and black pepper for about 4-5 minutes per side.
2. Transfer the beef shanks to a large Crockpot.
3. In the same skillet, sauté onion for about 3-4 minutes.
4. Add garlic and sauté for about 1 minute.
5. Place onion mixture over beef shanks and cover evenly with tomato paste.
6. With a kitchen string, tie the herbs sprigs.
7. Arrange tied sprigs over tomato paste and pour broth on top evenly.
8. Set the Crockpot on low and cook, covered, for about 8 hours.
9. Serve hot.

Lamb Recipes

Keto Lamb Barbacoa:

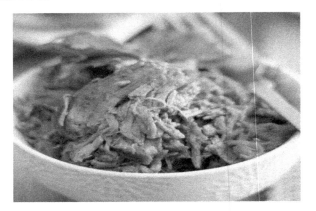

Serves: 10
Preparation Time: 10 minutes
Cooking Time: 6 hours
Macros per serving:
Calories: 492
Protein: 38 grams
Fat: 36 grams
Carbohydrates: 1.2 grams

What you'll need:

- 5 ½ pounds Boneless leg of lamb
- ¼ cup Dried mustard
- 2 tablespoons Himalayan salt
- 2 tablespoons Smoked paprika
- 1 tablespoon Grounded cumin
- 1 tablespoon Dried oregano
- 1 tablespoon Chipotle powder
- 1 cup Water

How to make it:

1. Take a small mixing bowl and add oregano, salt, paprika, cumin, and chipotle powder and mix everything properly.
2. Now coat the lamb with mustard and spread the spice you mixed in the bowl evenly on the lamb.
3. Place the marinated lamb in a slow cooker and add water to it.
4. Let it cook for six hours.
5. Shred the lamb with a fork after cooking.
6. Leave only one cup of water in the lamb and drain out the rest of the water.

Greek Lamb Roast:

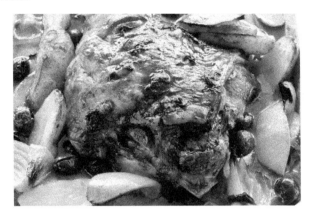

Serves: 2
Preparation Time: 10 minutes
Cooking Time: 4 hours
Macros per serving:
Calories: 443
Protein: 31 grams
Fat: 20 grams
Carbohydrates: 3 grams

What you'll need:

- 1 lemon
- 1 ¾ lb. leg of lamb, browned
- 2 teaspoons paprika
- 1 teaspoon dried oregano
- 1 cup chicken stock

How to make it:

1. Place lamb in Crock-Pot and add paprika, oregano, bay leaves (if desired), lemon juice and salt and pepper to taste.
2. Add the chicken stock and mix.
3. Cover and cook for 4 hours on high.
4. Use a spoon to scrape off undesired fat deposits to the meat.

Tasty Lamb Shoulders:

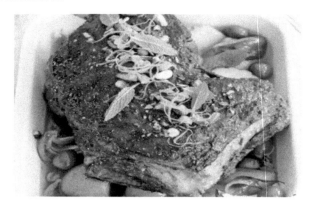

Serves: 4
Preparation Time: 10 minutes
Cooking Time: 4 hours
Macros per serving:
Calories: 441
Protein: 64.5 grams
Fat: 16.8 grams
Carbohydrates: 2.8 grams

What you'll need:

- 2 lbs. lamb shoulder
- ¼ cup beef broth
- ¼ cup fresh mint
- ¼ cup onion, chopped
- ¼ lb. carrots
- 2 tablespoons spice rub

How to make it:

1. Pour beef broth into the slow cooker.
2. Rub spice on all over lamb shoulder and place lamb shoulder into the slow cooker.
3. Add remaining ingredients into the slow cooker.
4. Cover and cook on high for 4 hours.
5. Shred the meat using a fork.
6. Serve and enjoy.

Island Lamb Stew:

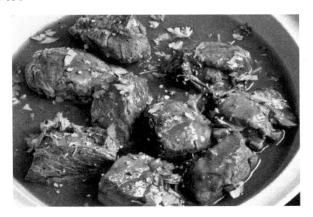

Serves: 4
Preparation Time: 15 minutes
Cooking Time: 8 hours
Macros per serving:
Calories: 352
Protein: 29.32 grams
Fat: 22.4 grams
Carbohydrates: 7.83 grams

What you'll need:

- 1 tablespoon butter
- 1 cup onion, sliced
- 1 pound lamb, diced
- 1 cup celery, sliced
- ¾ cup green pepper, chopped
- 1 tablespoon curry powder
- 1 can tomatoes
- Salt and pepper to taste

How to make it:

1. Set the Crockpot to high heat and add butter.
2. Sauté the onions for a minute then add the lamb.
3. Sear the lamb for 3 minutes.
4. Pour the remaining ingredients.
5. Close the lid and set the warmth to low.
6. Cook for 8 hours.

Basic Lamb Stew:

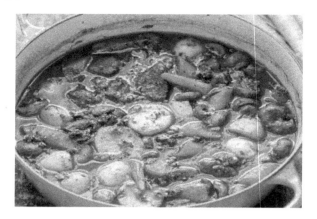

Serves: 2
Preparation Time: 5 minutes
Cooking Time: 3 hours
Macros per serving:
Calories: 380
Protein: 58 grams
Fat: 12 grams
Carbohydrates: 9 grams

What you'll need:

- 1 lb. boneless lamb stewing meat
- 8 oz. turnips, peeled and chopped
- 8 oz. mushrooms, sliced or quartered
- 14 oz. can of beef broth

How to make it:

1. Add all ingredients in a crock-pot. Also add seasonings: onion and garlic powder, salt and pepper to taste.
2. Cover and cook for 3 hours on high, or for 6 hours on low.
3. Check for seasoning additional} and add more if required.

Thyme Lamb Chops:

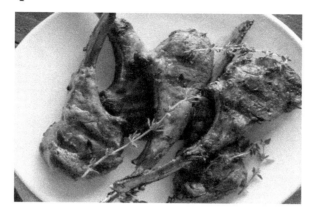

Serves: 2
Preparation Time: 10 minutes
Cooking Time: 6 hours
Macros per serving:
Calories: 257
Protein: 25.1 grams
Fat: 10.1 grams
Carbohydrates: 6.4 grams

What you'll need:

- 2 lamb shoulder chops, bone in
- ¼ cup fresh thyme
- 1 teaspoon garlic paste
- ½ cup red wine
- 1 cup beef broth
- Pepper
- Salt

How to make it:

1. Add all ingredients into the slow cooker and mix well.
2. Cover and cook on low for 6 hours.
3. Serve and enjoy.

Garlic Lamb Roast:

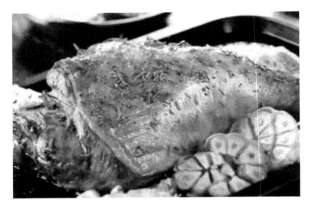

Serves: 2
Preparation Time: 10 minutes
Cooking Time: 10 hours
Macros per serving:
Calories: 435
Protein: 44 grams
Fat: 31 grams
Carbohydrates: 6 grams

What you'll need:

- 2 tablespoons coconut vinegar
- 1 teaspoon rosemary
- 1 leg of lamb
- 2 tablespoons Worcestershire sauce
- Desired veggies: chopped carrots, onions, and butternut squash

How to make it:

1. Put all ingredients in crock-pot. Add seasonings such as garlic, pepper, and salt to taste.
2. Cook on low for 6-10 hours or until the lamb is tender.

Garlic Herbed Lamb Chops:

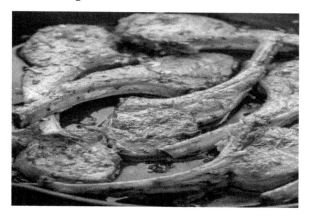

Serves: 4
Preparation Time: 10 minutes
Cooking Time: 4 hours
Macros per serving:
Calories: 656
Protein: 38.5 grams
Fat: 52.1 grams
Carbohydrates: 3.7 grams

What you'll need:

- 8 lamb loin chops
- 2 garlic cloves, minced
- 1/8 teaspoon black pepper
- ½ teaspoon garlic powder
- ½ teaspoon dried thyme
- 1 teaspoon dried oregano
- 1 medium onion, sliced
- ¼ teaspoon salt

How to make it:

1. In a small bowl, mix together oregano, garlic powder, thyme, pepper, and salt.
2. Rub herb mixture over the lamb chops.
3. Place lamb chops into the slow cooker.
4. Top lamb chops with garlic and sliced onion.
5. Cover and cook on low for 4 hours.
6. Serve and enjoy.

Tamil Attukal Paya Dish:

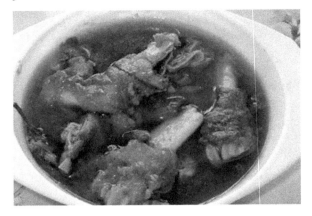

Serves: 10
Preparation Time: 10 minutes
Cooking Time: 10 hours
Macros per serving:
Calories: 184
Protein: 17.06 grams
Fat: 11.51 grams
Carbohydrates: 2.27 grams

What you'll need:

- 1 ½ pounds lamb fee, cut into chunks
- 1 onion, chopped
- 3 cloves of garlic
- 1 teaspoon black peppercorns
- 1-inch ginger, sliced thinly
- 1 can tomatoes
- 1 teaspoon coriander, ground
- ½ teaspoon cayenne pepper powder
- 1 bay leaf
- 4 cups water

How to make it:

1. Broil the lamb fee first in the oven for 10 minutes to add a roasted flavor on the soup.
2. Meanwhile, mix all other ingredients except the bay leaf and water in a food processor and pulse until fine.
3. Place the lamb feet in the Crockpot and pour over the sauce.
4. Add the bay leaf and water.
5. Cook on low for 10 hours.

Lamb Shanks with Tomatoes:

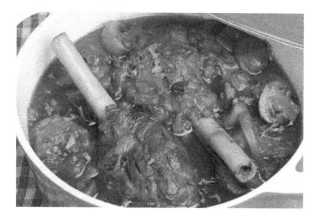

Serves: 2

Preparation Time: 15 minutes

Cooking Time: 8 hours

Macros per serving:

Calories: 397

Protein: 29 grams

Fat: 34 grams

Carbohydrates: 5 grams

What you'll need:

- 1/3 tablespoon tomato paste
- 1 x 400g tin diced tomatoes
- 1/3 tablespoon sundried tomato pesto
- 1/3 cup beef stock
- 2 lb. lamb shanks

How to make it:

1. Heat oil in a saucepan and cook onions until translucent. Add garlic and cook for 3 minutes.
2. Add ingredient and cook for an additional a pair of minutes, stirring.
3. Add diced tomatoes, sundried tomato pesto, and broth. Bring to a boil.
4. Put the lamb into the crock-pot and pour tomato sauce over.
5. Cook for 8 hours on low.

Delicious Balsamic Lamb Chops:

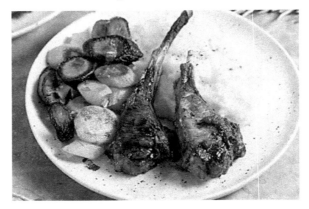

Serves: 6
Preparation Time: 10 minutes
Cooking Time: 6 hours
Macros per serving:
Calories: 496
Protein: 72.7 grams
Fat: 19.1 grams
Carbohydrates: 1.8 grams

What you'll need:

- 3.4 lbs. lamb chops, trimmed off
- ½ teaspoon ground black pepper
- 2 tablespoons rosemary
- 2 tablespoons balsamic vinegar
- 4 garlic cloves, minced
- 1 large onion, sliced
- ½ teaspoon salt

How to make it:

1. Add onion into the bottom of slow cooker.
2. Place lamb chops on top of onions, then and rosemary, vinegar, garlic, pepper, and salt.
3. Cover and cook on low for 6 hours.
4. Serve and enjoy.

Pot Roast Soup:

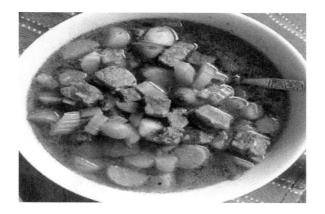

Serves: 4
Preparation Time: 15 minutes
Cooking Time: 8 hours
Macros per serving:
Calories: 211
Protein: 21.63 grams
Fat: 11.29 grams
Carbohydrates: 5.21 grams

What you'll need:

- 1 ¼ pound of meat stew
- 1 onion, diced
- 1 head cauliflower, diced
- 1 can diced tomatoes
- 1 Portobello mushroom, diced
- ¾ cup chicken stock
- 1 teaspoon dried basil
- 1 teaspoon dried oregano
- Salt and pepper to taste

How to make it:

1. Add all ingredients in the Crockpot.
2. Close the lid and cook on low for 8 hours or high for 5 hours.

Lamb Curry:

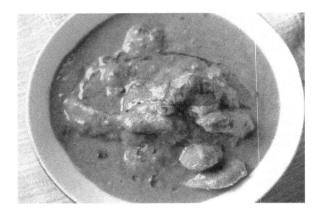

Serves: 2
Preparation Time: 25 minutes
Cooking Time: 8 hours
Macros per serving:
Calories: 554
Protein: 28 grams
Fat: 42 grams
Carbohydrates: 4 grams

What you'll need:

- 1 lamb shoulder
- 1 tablespoon curry powder
- 1 tablespoon ground coriander powder
- ½ cup tomato paste
- 1 x 400ml can coconut cream

How to make it:

1. Place lamb shoulder, roughly diced onions, roughly chopped garlic and ¼ cup water in crock-pot.
2. Cover and cook on low for 6-8 hours.
3. Put the meat aside and add the onions and garlic from crock-pot to ma frying pan.
4. Add curry powder and coriander powder. Cook until they are integrated.
5. Add tomato paste and cooked lamb meat. Cook for a further 5 minutes
6. Add coconut cream and simmer for 10 minutes on low heat.

Crockpot Ropa Vieja:

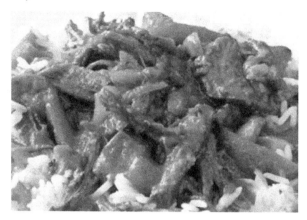

Serves: 8
Preparation Time: 20 minutes
Cooking Time: 8 hours
Macros per serving:
Calories: 277
Protein: 37.13 grams
Fat: 12.14 grams
Carbohydrates: 3.01 grams

What you'll need:

- 2 tablespoons coconut oil
- 3 pounds flanks steak
- 2 cloves of garlic, minced
- 3 peppers, sliced
- ¼ cup parsley, chopped
- ¼ cup cilantro, chopped
- 1 cup water
- 1 tablespoon white wine vinegar
- 2 cans of tomato sauce
- 1 tablespoon onion powder
- 1 tablespoon cumin powder
- 1 tablespoon oregano
- Salt to taste

How to make it:

1. In a skillet, heat oil and sear the flank steak for 3 minutes on each side. Set aside.
2. Place garlic, peppers, parsley, and cilantro in the Crockpot.
3. Add in the seared flank steak.
4. Pour in water, vinegar, and tomato sauce.
5. Add in the onion powder, cumin, and oregano.
6. Season with salt to taste.
7. Close the lid and cook on low for eight hours.

Ground Lamb Casserole:

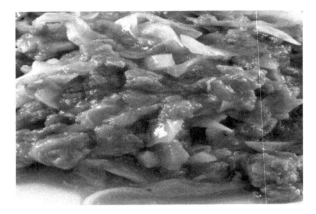

Serves: 2
Preparation Time: 5 minutes
Cooking Time: 8 hours
Macros per serving:
Calories: 295
Protein: 22 grams
Fat: 19 grams
Carbohydrates: 6 grams

What you'll need:

- 2 slices bacon, diced cooked crispy
- ½ lb. ground lamb
- 1/8 cup diced green bell pepper
- 2 cups thinly sliced cabbage
- 1 cup tomato sauce

How to make it:

1. Add the ground lamb, bacon, pepper, onion, and garlic to taste into the crock-pot.
2. Cover and cook for 6 hours in low.
3. Add the cabbage and tomato sauce to the pot, stir, then cook for another 2 hours.

Pork Recipes

Fabulous pork Casserole:

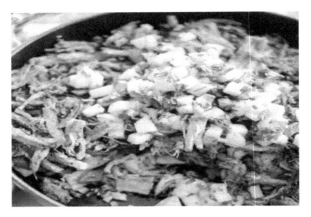

Serves: 8
Prep Time: 20minutes
Cook Time: 8hours 10 minutes
Macros per serving:
Calories: 296
Protein: 25.1grams
Fat: 17.6grams
Carbohydrates: 11grams

What you'll need:

- 1 tablespoon coconut oil
- 1 pound ground pork
- 1 onion, chopped
- 2 garlic cloves, minced
- ½ teaspoon red pepper flakes
- Salt, to taste
- 5 ounces fresh spinach
- 12 organic eggs
- 1 cup unsweetened coconut oil
- 1 pound butternut squash, peeled, seeded and chopped

How to make it:

1. Grease a crockpot
2. In a skillet, heat coconut oil and cook the pork for about 4-5 minutes
3. Stir in onion, garlic, red pepper flakes, and salt and cook for about 2-3 minutes.
4. Stir in spinach and cook for regarding a pair of minutes.
5. Remove from heat and keep aside to chill slightly.
6. To a bowl, add almond milk and eggs and beat well.
7. In the bottom of prepared crockpot, place squash, followed by pork mixture and egg mixture.
8. Set the crockpot on low and cook, covered, for about 6-8 hours.
9. Cut into 8 equal sized wedges and serve.

Chili Pulled Pork Tacos:

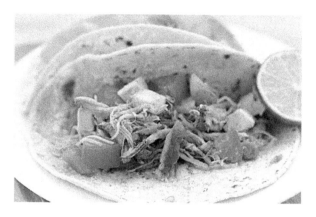

Serves: 10
Preparation Time: 10-15 minutes
Cooking Time: 8 hours
Macros per serving:
Calories: 159.8
Protein: 20.6 grams
Fat: 7 grams
Carbohydrates: 2.7 grams

What you'll need:

- 4 ½ pounds Pork meet butt or shoulder
- 1 ½ teaspoons Cumin grounded
- 2 tablespoons Chili powder
- ½ teaspoon Oregano grounded
- ½ cup Broth
- ¼ teaspoon Red pepper flakes
- 1 Bay leaf
- A pinch Grounded cloves
- Salt to taste

How to make it:

1. Combine salt, oregano, chili powder, cumin, cloves and pepper flakes in medium bowl.
2. Clean the pork and rub the spice mixture on the pork meet.
3. Keep it in the fridge for about 2 hours and let it get marinated properly.
4. Now keep ready your Crockpot slow cooker and put the marinated meet to it.
5. Add the broth and Bay leaf.
6. Cook it about 8 hours by setting on slow cooking.
7. Once cooking is over, place the cooked meet on a cutting board and by using two forks, and shred the meat.
8. Serve it hot.

Root Beer Pulled Pork:

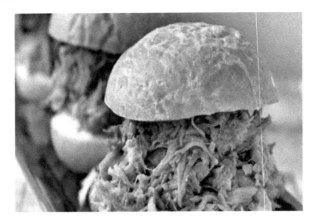

Serves: 2
Preparation Time: 15 minutes
Cooking Time: 8 hours
Macros per serving:
Calories: 345
Protein: 18.6 grams
Fat: 27.8 grams
Carbohydrates: 4.3 grams

What you'll need:

- 1 (12 oz.)can or bottle root beer
- 1 (4 oz.) bottle liquid smoke flavoring, or to taste
- 1 (4 lb.)pork shoulder roast

How to make it:

1. Prepare the seasoning: salt, pepper, and garlic to taste.
2. Rub seasoning on all sides of pork.
3. Put the pork with all other ingredients in the Crockpot.
4. Cook for 8 hours on low.

Cuban Pulled Pork:

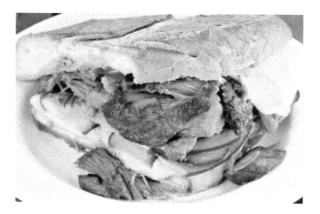

Serves: 6
Preparation Time: 10 minutes
Cooking Time: 8 hours
Macros per serving:
Calories: 461
Protein: 35.9 grams
Fat: 32.8 grams
Carbohydrates: 4.1 grams

What you'll need:

- 2 lbs. pork shoulder, cut into 4" pieces
- 2 tablespoons fresh cilantro, chopped
- ¼ teaspoon red pepper flakes
- 1 ½ teaspoons paprika
- 1 ½ teaspoons cumin
- 1 ½ teaspoon chili powder
- 1 tablespoon dry oregano
- ¼ cup oregano juice
- 3 garlic cloves, chopped
- 1 tablespoon lime juice
- 1 small onion, chopped
- ½ teaspoon salt

How to make it:

1. Add all ingredients into the slow cooker and stir well to mix.
2. Cover and cook on low for 8 hours.
3. Shred meat using a fork and serve.

Pork Stew with Oyster Mushrooms:

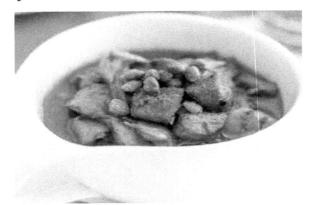

Serves: 4
Preparation Time: 15 minutes
Cooking Time: 6 hours
Macros per serving:
Calories: 374
Protein: 50.4 grams
Fat: 48.9 grams
Carbohydrates: 23.5 grams

What you'll need:

- 2 tablespoons coconut oil
- 1 onion, chopped
- 1 clove of garlic, chopped
- 2 pounds pork loin
- Salt and pepper to taste
- 2 tablespoons dried mustard
- 2 tablespoons dried oregano
- ½ teaspoon nutmeg powder
- 1 ½ cups bone broth
- 2 tablespoons white wine vinegar
- 2 pounds oyster mushroom
- ¼ cup coconut milk
- 3 tablespoons capers

How to make it:

1. Heat the Crockpot to high and add coconut oil.
2. Sauté the onion and garlic for two minutes and add in the pork loin. Sear and season with salt and pepper to taste.
3. Stir in the mustard, oregano, and nutmeg.
4. Pour in the bone broth and white wine vinegar
5. Add in the mushrooms.
6. Close the lid and adjust the cooking temperature to low.
7. Cook for 6 hours
8. Ten minutes before the cooking time, add in the coconut milk and capers.

Beamless Pork Chili:

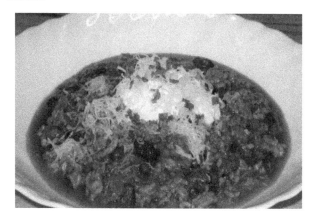

Serves: 8
Preparation Time: 20 minutes
Cooking Time: 6 hours 10 minutes
Macros per serving:
Calories: 283
Protein: 20.4 grams
Fat: 17.3 grams
Carbohydrates: 9 grams

What you'll need:

- 2 medium green bell peppers, seeded and chopped
- 1 medium yellow onion, chopped
- ½ tablespoon olive oil
- 2 pounds lean ground pork
- Salt and freshly ground black pepper, to taste
- 8 thick bacon slices, chopped
- 2 cups tomatoes, chopped
- 1 ½ teaspoon ground cumin
- 2 teaspoons red chili powder
- ½ teaspoon cayenne pepper
- ¾ cup sugar-free tomato paste

How to make it:

1. In the bottom of a Crockpot, place bell pepper and onion.
2. In a large skillet, heat oil over medium-high heat and cook pork with salt and black pepper for about 4-5 minutes.
3. Transfer the pork into Crockpot.
4. In the same skillet, add bacon and cook for 4-5 minutes.
5. Place cooked bacon and tomatoes over pork and sprinkle evenly with spices.
6. Pour tomato paste on top evenly.
7. Set the Crockpot on low and cook, covered, for about 6 hours.

Pork Roast with Sugarless Chimichurri Sauce:

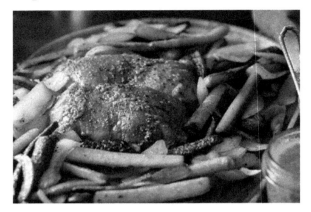

Serves: 12
Preparation Time: 30 minutes
Cooking Time: 6 hours
Macros per serving:
Calories: 167
Protein: 17 grams
Fat: 8 grams
Carbohydrates: 5 grams

What you'll need:

- 3 pounds Pork roast boneless
- 4 tablespoons Extra virgin olive oil
- 1 pound Carrots trimmed and quartered lengthwise
- Sweet onion thickly sliced
- Real salt to taste
- Chimichurri sauce (prepare as per the recipe)

How to make it:

1. Place the pork roasted in a pot. Add 2 tablespoons of the olive oil over the roast and sprinkle it with salt and pepper.
2. Cover and cook on high for 6 hours. In slow cooking, cook it about 12 hours.
3. After 4 hours of cooking, add the onions and carrots around the roast.
4. Cook the roast, carrots, and onions for 2 hours until you can easily pull apart the pork and the carrots become soft.
5. Place the roast, carrots, and onion on serving platter and drizzle with sauce.
6. Serve with extra sauce as per you like.

For Chimichurri Sauce:

- 1 cup Basil fresh
- 3 garlic clove
- 2 tablespoons lemon juice
- ½ cup olive oil, extra virgin
- ¼ teaspoon black pepper
- ¼ teaspoon cayenne pepper
- 1 teaspoon salt

How to make it:

1. In a food processor, combine all the ingredients.
2. Continue blending until the basil becomes small and even.
3. Your sauce is ready to sprinkle on the dish.

Creamy Onion Pork Chops:

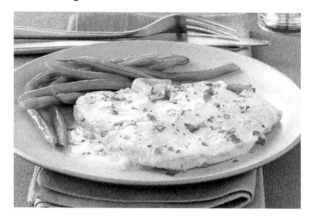

Serves: 2
Preparation Time: 10 minutes
Cooking Time: 7 hours
Macros per serving:
Calories: 931.7
Protein: 84.4 grams
Fat: 61.5 grams
Carbohydrates: 5 grams

What you'll need:

- 4 pork chops, browned
- 1 chicken bouillon cubes
- ½ large onion ¼ -inch slices
- 4 oz. sour cream
- 1/8 cup olive oil

How to make it:

1. Put the pork chops in a crock-pot and place onions on top.
2. Dissolve bouillon in hot water and pour in the Crockpot.
3. Cook for 7 to 8 hours on low.
4. When cooked thoroughly, add sour cream into the pot. Turn to high and cook further for about 30 minutes.

Asian Pulled Pork:

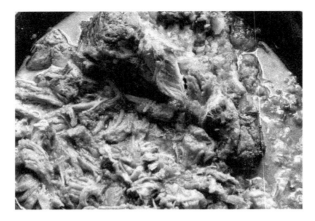

Serves: 6
Preparation Time: 10 minutes
Cooking Time: 8 hours 30 minutes
Macros per serving:
Calories: 334
Protein: 43.3 grams
Fat: 14.3 grams
Carbohydrates: 4.5 grams

What you'll need:

- 2 lbs. pork roasted
- 2 tablespoons oyster sauce
- 1 teaspoon garlic, minced
- 1 tablespoon Worcestershire sauce
- ¼ cups coconut aminos
- 1 onion, sliced
- 1 cup water

How to make it:

1. Spray slow cooker from inside with cooking spray.
2. Pour water into the slow cooker.
3. Place roast into the slow cooker.
4. Place sliced onion around the roast.
5. Cover and cook on low for 8 hours.
6. Shred the meat using a fork.
7. In a small bowl, combine together coconut aminos, oyster sauce, garlic, and Worcestershire sauce.
8. Pour coconut aminos mixture over shredded pork and stir well and cook for 30 minutes more.
9. Serve and enjoy.

Easy Pork Luau:

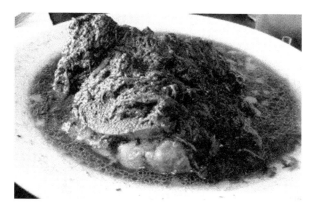

Serves: 10
Preparation Time: 15 minutes
Cooking Time: 7 hours
Macros per serving:
Calories: 182
Protein: 14 grams
Fat: 13 grams
Carbohydrates: 2 grams

What you'll need:

- 4 slices of smoked bacon
- 5 cloves of garlic, minced
- 3 pounds pork roast shoulder
- 1 ½ tablespoon Hawaiian black lava sea salt or ordinary salt
- 2 tablespoons liquid smoke

How to make it:

1. Set the Crockpot to high setting and place the raw bacon slices.
2. Sprinkle minced garlic over the bacon.
3. Using a knife, poke holes through the pork roast to allow heat and the sauce to seep into the meat.
4. Rub salt all over the pork. Place the pork inside the Crockpot.
5. Add the liquid smoke.
6. Adjust the cooking setting and cook on low for 8 hours.
7. Shred the meat with the fork.

Traditional Burmese Pork Curry:

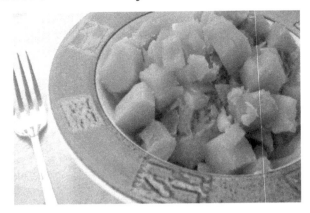

Serves: 6
Preparation Time: 20 minutes
Cooking Time: 8 hours
Macros per serving:
Calories: 272
Protein: 41.2 grams
Fat: 5.7 grams
Carbohydrates: 13.3 grams

What you'll need:

- 4 garlic cloves, minced
- 1 teaspoon fresh ginger, grated finely
- 1 tablespoon fish sauce
- 1 tablespoon soy sauce
- 2 teaspoons paprika
- 1 teaspoon ground cumin
- 1 teaspoon ground turmeric
- 2 pounds boneless pork chops
- 2 medium onions, chopped
- 1 pound winter squash, cubed

How to make it:

1. In a bowl, add garlic, ginger, fish sauce, soy sauce, and spices and mix well.
2. In a large Crockpot, place pork chops and top evenly with spice mixture.
3. Place onion on top, evenly, followed by squash cubes.
4. Set the Crockpot on low and cook, covered, for about 7-8 hours.
5. Serve hot.

Pulled Pork with BBQ Sauce:

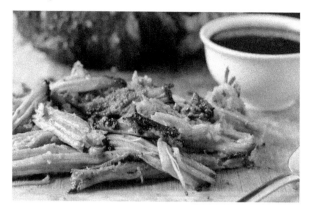

Serves: 2
Preparation Time: 15 minutes
Cooking Time: 6 hours
Macros per serving:
Calories: 497
Protein: 35 grams
Fat: 36.6 grams
Carbohydrates: 3.8 grams

What you'll need:

- 1/3 cup spray chocolate BBQ sauce
- 3.5 kg pork shoulder, boneless, skin scored
- 1 tablespoon paprika
- 3 bay leaves

How to make it:

1. Prepare the seasons: one large white onion, salt, and pepper to taste, to be mixed with paprika.
2. Rub the seasonings with the pork. Put in the crock-pot add bay leaves on top.
3. Cover and cook for 5 hours on high.
4. When cooked and tender. Add the BBQ sauce and cook for an additional hour.

Simple Pork Tenderloin:

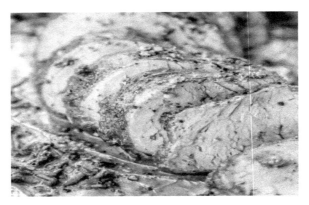

Serves: 6
Preparation Time: 10 minutes
Cooking Time: 8 hours 5 minutes
Macros per serving:
Calories: 294
Protein: 51.3 grams
Fat: 7.3 grams
Carbohydrates: 2.3 grams

What you'll need:

- 2 ½ lbs. pork tenderloin
- 2 tablespoons Worcestershire sauce
- 1 teaspoon oregano
- 1 teaspoon paprika
- 2 teaspoons cumin
- 2 garlic cloves, minced
- 2 cups chicken broth
- Pepper
- Salt

How to make it:

1. Add all ingredients to the slow cooker.
2. Cover and cook on low for 8 hours.
3. Shred the meat using a fork.
4. Place shredded meat on a baking tray and broil for 5 minutes.
5. Serve and enjoy.

Crockpot Pork Carnitas:

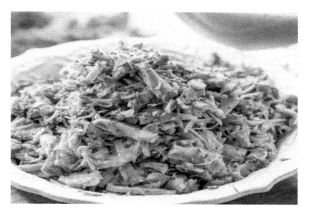

Serves: 10
Preparation Time: 10 minutes
Cooking Time: 6 hours
Macros per serving:
Calories: 155
Protein: 25.96 grams
Fat: 3.99 grams
Carbohydrates: 2.29 grams

What you'll need:

- 2 ½ pounds boneless pork shoulder
- 5 cloves of garlic, minced
- 2 teaspoons ground cumin
- 2 teaspoons oregano
- 1 tablespoon sherry vinegar
- Salt and pepper to taste
- 1 onion, quartered
- 4 bay leaves

How to make it:

1. Place pork, garlic, cumin, oregano, and sherry vinegar in the Crockpot. Season with salt and pepper.
2. Add the onions and bay leaves.
3. Cover the Crockpot and set on low temperature.
4. Cook for six hours.
5. Once done, shred the meat using the fork.

Chinese Pulled Pork:

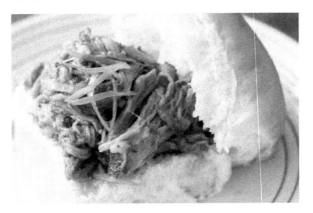

Serves: 2
Preparation Time: 10 minutes
Cooking Time: 7 hours
Macros per serving:
Calories: 459
Protein: 30 grams
Fat: 35 grams
Carbohydrates: 3 grams

What you'll need:

- 1 1/3 tablespoons sugar-free tomato sauce
- 1/3 tablespoon tomato paste
- 1/3 teaspoon Smoked paprika
- 12 oz. pork shoulder or loin
- 1/3 cup chicken broth

How to make it:

1. Prepare the seasoning: garlic, ginger, soy sauce and sweetener to taste, together with tomato paste, tomato sauce, and paprika.
2. Put the seasoning in the chicken broth and mix thoroughly.
3. Pour the mixture in the pork placed in the bottom of a Crockpot.
4. Cover and cook for 7 hours on low.

Seafood Recipes

Nutritious Salmon Stew:

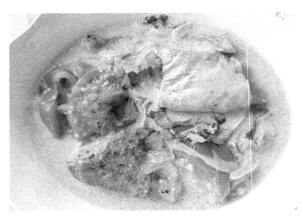

Serves: 4

Preparation Time: 15 minutes

Cooking Time: 6 hours

Macros per serving:

Calories: 159

Protein: 23.4 grams

Fat: 10.7 grams

Carbohydrates: 7.2 grams

What you'll need:

- 1 pound salmon fillet, cubed
- 1 tablespoon coconut oil
- 1 medium yellow onion, chopped
- 1 garlic clove, minced
- 1 zucchini, sliced
- 1 green bell pepper, seeded and cubed
- ½ cup tomatoes, chopped
- ½ homemade fish broth
- ¼ teaspoon dried oregano
- ¼ teaspoon dried basil
- Salt and freshly ground black pepper, to taste

How to make it:

1. In a large Crockpot, add all ingredients and mix.
2. Set the Crockpot on low and cook, covered, for about 4-6 hours.
3. Serve hot.

Shrimp Scampi:

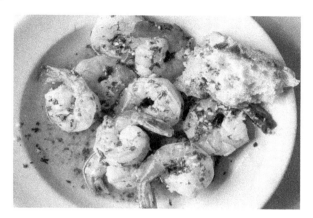

Serves: 2
Preparation Time: 5 minutes
Cooking Time: 2 hours 30 minutes
Macros per serving:
Calories: 156
Protein: 23.3 grams
Fat: 14.7 grams
Carbohydrates: 2 grams

What you'll need:

- ½ lb. raw shrimp, peeled and deveined
- 1/8 cup chicken broth
- 1 tablespoon butter
- ½ tablespoon lemon juice
- ¼ cup white cooking wine

How to make it:

1. Combine everything in the Crockpot. Add salt and pepper (and red pepper flakes if desired) to taste.
2. Cover and cook for 2.5 hours on low.

Tuna and White Beans:

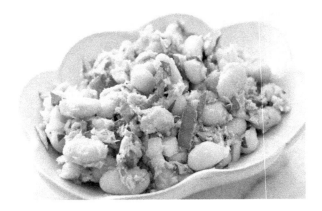

Serves: 4
Preparation Time: 10 minutes
Cooking Time: 5 hours 15 minutes
Macros per serving:
Calories: 764
Protein: 62.84 grams
Fat: 25.43 grams
Carbohydrates: 12.05 grams

What you'll need:

- 4 tablespoon olive oil
- 1 clove of garlic, minced
- 6 cups water
- 1 pound white beans, soaked overnight and drained
- 2 cups chopped tomatoes
- 3 cans white tuna, drained and flaked
- 2 sprigs of basil
- Salt and pepper to taste

How to make it:

1. Set the Crockpot to high heat and add oil.
2. Sauté the garlic for 2 minutes and add water.
3. Stir in the beans. Close the lid and cook on high for five hours.
4. Add in the tomatoes, tuna, and basil.
5. Season with salt and pepper to taste.
6. Continue cooking on high for 15 minutes.

Mustard-Crusted Salmon:

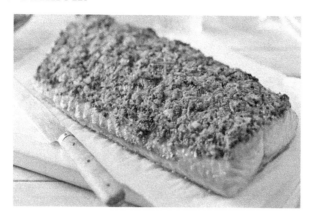

Serves: 4
Preparation Time: 3 minutes
Cooking Time: 4 hours
Macros per serving:
Calories: 74
Protein: 25.9 grams
Fat: 13.8 grams
Carbohydrates: 4.2 grams

What you'll need:

- 4 pieces salmon fillets
- Salt and pepper to taste
- 2 teaspoons lemon juice
- 2 tablespoons stone-ground mustard
- ¼ cup full sour cream

How to make it:

1. Season salmon fillet with salt and pepper to style. Sprinkle with lemon juice.
2. Rub the stone-ground mustard all over the fillets.
3. Place inside the Crockpot and cook on high for 2 hours or on low for 4 hours.
4. An hour before the cooking time, pour in the sour cream on top of the fish.
5. Continue cooking until the fish becomes flaky.

Entrée Cod Stew:

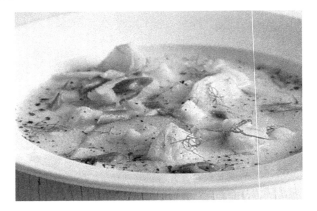

Serves: 4
Preparation Time: 20 minutes
Cooking Time: 2 hours
Macros per serving:
Calories: 173
Protein: 28.6 grams
Fat: 1.9 grams
Carbohydrates: 10.9 grams

What you'll need:

- 1 (28-ounce) can sugar-free diced tomatoes
- ¼ cup homemade fish broth
- 1 bell pepper, seeded and chopped
- 1 zucchini, spiralized with blade C
- 1 medium yellow onion, chopped
- 3 garlic cloves, minced
- 3 teaspoons ground cumin
- ¼ teaspoon red pepper flakes
- Salt and freshly ground black pepper, to taste
- 1 pound cod fillets

How to make it:

1. In a large Crockpot, add all ingredients except cod and mix.
2. Place cod fillets on top.
3. Set the Crockpot on high and cook covered, for about 1-2 hours.
4. Serve hot.

Braised Squid with Tomatoes and Fennel:

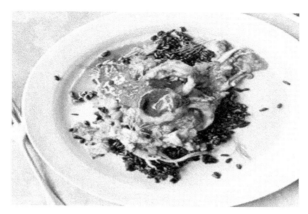

Serves: 2
Preparation Time: 20 minutes
Cooking Time: 4 hours
Macros per serving:
Calories: 210
Protein: 29 grams
Fat: 25 grams
Carbohydrates: 6 grams

What you'll need:

- 1 ½ cups clam juice
- 1 can plum tomatoes
- ½ fennel bulb, minced
- 3 tablespoons all-purpose flour
- 1 lb. squid in 1 –inch pieces

How to make it:

1. Add chopped onions, fennel and garlic to the flameproof insert of a Crockpot and cook on a stove in medium heat for about 5 minutes.
2. Whisk in flour and tomato paste until fully mixed. Add the clam juice, tomatoes, 1 teaspoon salt and pepper. Boil for about 2 minutes.
3. Transfer to the Crockpot, cover and cook for hours on low.
4. Uncover, add the squid and mix well. Cook for another 1 hour.

Crockpot Swordfish Steaks:

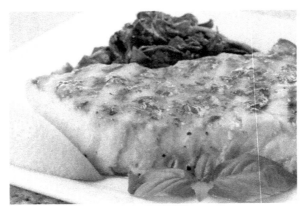

Serves: 6
Preparation Time: 10 minutes
Cooking Time: 2 hours
Macros per serving:
Calories: 659
Protein: 46.59 grams
Fat: 50.78 grams
Carbohydrates: 1.63 grams

What you'll need:

- 6 swordfish steaks
- ½ cup olive oil
- ¼ cup lemon juice
- ½ teaspoon Worcestershire sauce
- ¼ teaspoon black pepper
- 1 teaspoon cayenne pepper powder
- ¼ teaspoon paprika

How to make it:

1. Place the swordfish steaks in the Crockpot.
2. Pour the other ingredients over the swordfish steaks.
3. Close the lid and cook on high for two hours.

Five- Spice Tilapia:

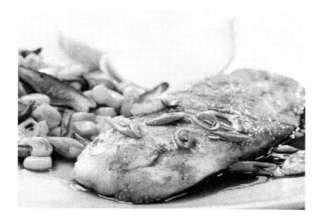

Serves: 4
Preparation Time: 3 minutes
Cooking Time: 5 hours
Macros per serving:
Calories: 153
Protein: 25.8 grams
Fat: 5.6 grams
Carbohydrates: 0.9 grams

What you'll need:

- 4 Italian fillets
- 1 teaspoon Chinese five-spice powder
- 1 tablespoon sesame oil
- ¼ cup gluten-free soy sauce
- 3 scallions, thinly sliced

How to make it:

1. Season the tilapia fillets with the Chinese five-spice powder.
2. Place sesame oil in the Crockpot and arrange the fish on top.
3. Cook on high for 2 hours and on low for 4 hours.
4. Halfway through the cooking time, flip the fish to slightly brown the other side.
5. Once cooking time is done, add the soy sauce and scallion and continue cooking for another hour.

South-Indian Cod Curry:

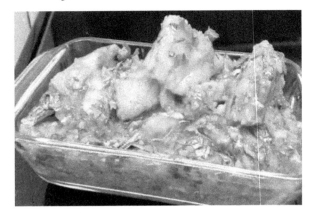

Serves: 8
Preparation Time: 20 minutes
Cooking Time: 2 hours 20 minutes
Macros per serving:
Calories: 369
Protein: 28.7 grams
Fat: 25.5 grams
Carbohydrates: 9.2 grams

What you'll need:

- ½ cup unsweetened coconut flakes
- ½ small yellow onion, chopped roughly
- ½ teaspoon fresh turmeric, peeled and chopped roughly
- ½ teaspoon fresh ginger, peeled and chopped roughly
- 2 garlic cloves, sliced thinly
- 2 Serrano chilies, sliced
- 1 teaspoon coriander seeds
- 2 tablespoons tamarind paste
- 1 teaspoon ground cumin
- ¼ teaspoon fenugreek seeds
- 1 tablespoon mild curry powder
- Salt, to taste
- 2 (13 ½ -ounce) cans unsweetened coconut milk
- 2 pounds cod fillets, cut into 2-3 inch pieces

How to make it:

1. In a food processor, add all ingredients except coconut milk and cod and pulse until smooth.
2. Transfer the paste into a pan with coconut milk and bring to a boil.
3. Transfer coconut mixture into a Crockpot.
4. Set the Crockpot on high and cook covered, for about 2 hours.
5. Season cod fillets with a little salt.
6. Uncover the Crockpot and submerge cod in curry sauce.
7. Set the Crockpot on low and cook, covered, for about 20 minutes.
8. Serve hot.

Fish Curry with Coconut and Spinach:

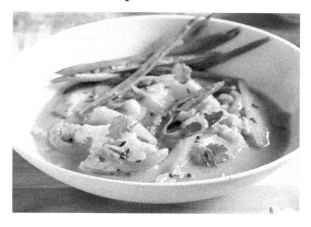

Serves: 2
Preparation Time: 10 minutes
Cooking Time: 4 hours
Macros per serving:
Calories: 314
Protein: 33.4 grams
Fat: 18.5 grams
Carbohydrates: 3.6 grams

What you'll need:

- 2/3 tablespoon curry paste of choice
- ½ cups coconut cream
- ¾ lb. firm white fish cut into cubes
- ½ lb. spinach washed and sliced

How to make it:

1. Put all the ingredients in the Crockpot except the spinach. Add ½ cup of water.
2. Cook for 3 hours on low.
3. Add the spinach and cook for another 1 hour to wilt the spinach.

Rustic Fish and Tomatoes:

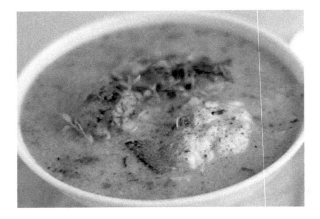

Serves: 4
Preparation Time: 10 minutes
Cooking Time: 3 hours
Macros per serving:
Calories: 103
Protein: 18.68 grams
Fat: 0.76 grams
Carbohydrates: 5.3 grams

What you'll need:

- 1 pound cod fillet
- 3 cloves of garlic, minced
- 1 onion, sliced
- 1 bell pepper, sliced
- 1 tablespoon rosemary
- 1 can diced tomatoes
- ¼ teaspoon red pepper flakes
- ¼ cup broth
- Salt and pepper to taste

How to make it:

1. Place all ingredients in the Crockpot and stir to mix well.
2. Cook on low for 3 hours or high for 30 minutes.

Prosciutto-Wrapped Scallops:

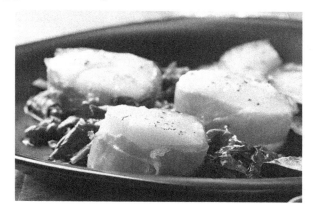

Serves: 4
Preparation Time: 3 minutes
Cooking Time: 3 hours
Macros per serving:
Calories: 113
Protein: 15.9 grams
Fat: 8 grams
Carbohydrates: 5 grams

What you'll need:

- 12 large scallops, rinsed and patted dry
- Salt and pepper to taste
- 1 ¼ ounces prosciutto, cut into 12 long strips
- 1 tablespoon extra-virgin olive oil
- 1 tablespoon lemon juice

How to make it:

1. Sprinkle individual scallops with salt and pepper to taste.
2. Wrap prosciutto around the scallops. Set aside.
3. Add oil in Crockpot and arrange on top the bacon-wrapped scallops.
4. Pour over the lemon juice.
5. Cook on low for 1 hour or on high for 3 hours.
6. Halfway through the cooking time, flip the scallops.
7. Continue cooking until scallops are done.

Thai Halibut Curry:

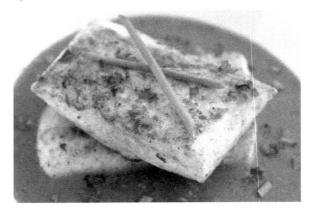

Serves: 4
Preparation Time: 15 minutes
Cooking Time: 2 hours
Macros per serving:
Calories: 365
Protein: 33.7 grams
Fat: 22.8 grams
Carbohydrates: 8.6 grams

What you'll need:

- 1 tablespoon olive oil
- 1 tablespoon Thai red curry paste
- 1 onion, sliced
- 1 cup coconut milk
- 1 pound skinless halibut, cut into chunks
- 7 ounces fresh green beans, trimmed
- Salt and freshly ground black pepper, to taste

How to make it:

1. In a large Crockpot, heat oil and sauté curry paste for about 1 minute.
2. Add onion and cook for about 5 minutes.
3. Add remaining ingredients and stir to combine
4. Set the Crockpot on low and cook, covered, for about 1 ½ -2 hours.
5. Serve hot.

Lobster Bisque:

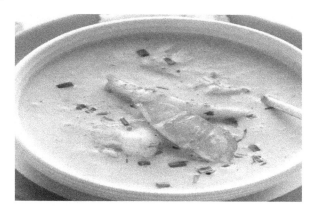

Serves: 2
Preparation Time: 20 minutes
Cooking Time: 6 hours
Macros per serving:
Calories: 400
Protein: 23 grams
Fat: 30 grams
Carbohydrates: 7 grams

What you'll need:

- 1 1/3 lobster tails, fan parts cut out
- 2/3 teaspoon Worcestershire sauce
- 2 tablespoons tomato paste
- 2/3 cup lobster stock
- 2/3 cup heavy cream

How to make it:

1. Enhance the broth: slowly add broth to an onion-garlic sauté.
2. Add this broth and all the other ingredients except the heavy cream in the crock-pot, including desired slices to taste (paprika, thyme, black pepper)
3. Cover and cook on low for 6 hours.

Salmon with lime Butter:

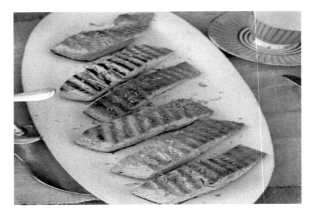

Serves: 4
Preparation Time: 3 minutes
Cooking Time: 4 hours
Macros per serving:
Calories: 206
Protein: 23.7 grams
Fat: 15.2 grams
Carbohydrates: 1.8 grams

What you'll need:

- 1-pound salmon fillet cut into 4 portions
- 1 tablespoon butter, melted
- Salt and pepper to taste
- 2 tablespoons lime juice
- ½ teaspoon lime zest, grated

How to make it:

1. Add all ingredients in the Crockpot.
2. Close the lid.
3. Cook on high for 2 hours and on low for 4 hours.

Vegetarian Recipes

Delicious Vegetable Medley:

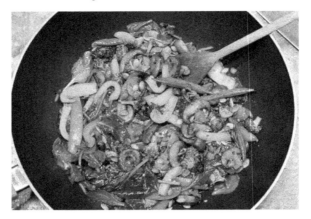

Serves: 8
Preparation Time: 10 minutes
Cooking Time: 6 hours
Macros per serving:
Calories: 29
Protein: 1.6 grams
Fat: 0.2 grams
Carbohydrates: 6.5 grams

What you'll need:

- 2 cups mushrooms, sliced
- 14 oz. can tomatoes, diced
- 1 zucchini, chopped
- 1 bell pepper, chopped
- 1 onion, chopped
- ½ teaspoon oregano
- ¼ teaspoon garlic powder
- 1/8 teaspoon black pepper

How to make it:

1. Add all ingredients to the slow cookware and stir well.
2. Cover and cook on low for 6 hours.
3. Stir well and serve.

Slow Cooker Mushroom Sauté:

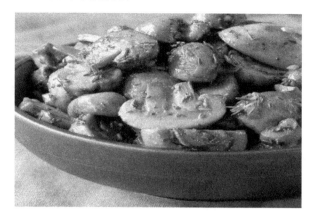

Serves: 4
Preparation Time: 5 minutes
Cooking Time: 1 hour 30 minutes
Macros per serving:
Calories: 94
Protein: 2.3 grams
Fat: 1.4 grams
Carbohydrates: 5.3 grams

What you'll need:

- 1 pound Button mushrooms, sliced
- 1 tablespoon Butter
- ½ tablespoon Olive oil
- ½ tablespoon Balsamic vinegar
- 1/8 tablespoon Oregano, dried
- 1 Clove garlic, minced
- ¼ cup Water
- Salt to taste
- Pepper to taste

How to make it:

1. In a massive frying pan, soften butter with oil.
2. Add water, mushroom, garlic, oregano, vinegar, salt and sauté for about 5 minutes.
3. Then transfer all these to your Crockpot slow cooker.
4. Set slow cooking for about 1 hour 30 minutes, until mushroom becomes tender.
5. Stir occasionally.
6. Serve hot.

Italian Veggie Frittata:

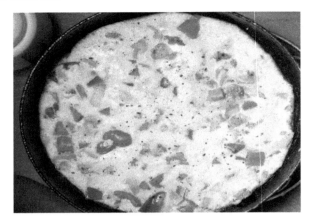

Serves: 4
Preparation Time: 20 minutes
Cooking Time: 2 hours
Macros per serving:
Calories: 128
Protein: 10.1 grams
Fat: 8.7 grams
Carbohydrates: 3.2 grams

What you'll need:

- 1 teaspoon butter
- 4 ounces fresh mushrooms, sliced
- ¼ cup cherry tomatoes, sliced
- ¼ cup fresh kale, trimmed and chopped
- 2 scallions, sliced
- 6 organic eggs
- 1 tablespoon parmesan cheese, shredded
- 2 teaspoons Italian seasoning
- Salt and freshly ground black pepper, to taste

How to make it:

1. Grease a Crockpot.
2. In a large skillet, melt butter over medium heat and sauté mushrooms, tomatoes, kale, and scallions for about 4-5 minute.
3. Transfer the veggie mixture into prepared Crockpot.
4. In a bowl, add remaining ingredients and beat till well combined.
5. Pour egg mixture over mixture evenly and stir gently to combine.
6. Set the Crockpot on high and cook, covered, for about 1-2 hours.
7. Cut into 4 equal sized wedges and serve.

Veggie-Noodle Soup:

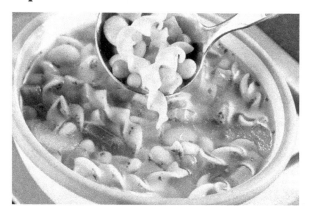

Serves: 2
Preparation Time: 10 minutes
Cooking Time: 8 hours
Macros per serving:
Calories: 56
Protein: 3 grams
Fat: 0.5 grams
Carbohydrates: 0.5 grams

What you'll need:

- ½ cup chopped carrots, chopped
- ½ cup chopped celery, chopped
- 1 teaspoon Italian seasoning
- 7 oz. zucchini, cut spiral
- 2 cups spinach leaves, chopped

How to make it:

1. Except for the zucchini and spinach, add all the ingredients to the Crockpot.
2. Add 3 cups of water.
3. Add ½ cup of chopped onion and garlic, 1/8 teaspoon of salt and pepper and desired spices such as thyme and bay leaves if desired.
4. Cover and cook for 8 hours on low.
5. Add the zucchini and spinach at the last 10 minutes of cooking.

Spicy Eggplant with Red pepper and Parsley:

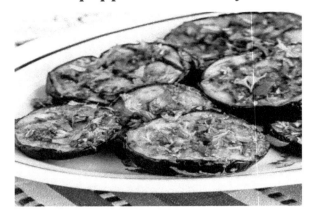

Serves: 4
Preparation Time: 3 minutes
Cooking Time: 3 hours
Macros per serving:
Calories: 52
Protein: 1.8 grams
Fat: 0.31 grams
Carbohydrates: 11.67 grams

What you'll need:

- 1 large eggplant, sliced
- 2 tablespoons parsley, chopped
- 1 big red bell pepper, chopped
- Salt and pepper to taste
- 2 tablespoons balsamic vinegar

How to make it:

1. Place all ingredients in a mixing bowl.
2. Toss to coat ingredients
3. Place in the Crockpot and cook on low for 3 hours on high for 1 hour.

Healthy Brussels sprouts:

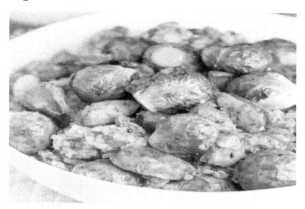

Serves: 6
Preparation Time: 10 minutes
Cooking Time: 2 hours 30 minutes
Macros per serving:
Calories: 74
Protein: 3.9 grams
Fat: 3 grams
Carbohydrates: 10 grams

What you'll need:

- 2 lbs. Brussels sprouts, cut in half
- 2 tablespoons olive oil
- 1/3 cup vinegar
- 1 garlic clove, minced
- 2 tablespoons chives, sliced
- Pepper
- Salt

How to make it:

1. Add all ingredients to the slow cookware and blend well.
2. Cover and cook on high for two hours half-hour.
3. Stir well and serve.

Crockpot Cauliflower Side Dish:

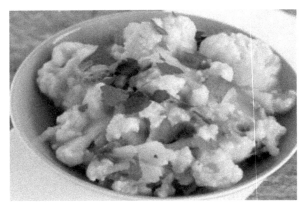

Serves: 12

Preparation Time: 20 minutes

Cooking Time: 1 hour 30 minutes -2hours

Macros per serving:

Calories: 276

Protein: 10 grams

Fat: 18 grams

Carbohydrates: 9.7 grams

What you'll need:

- 16 ounces Fresh cauliflower
- 8 ounces Sour cream
- 3 teaspoons Chicken bouillon granules
- 1 ½ cups Cheddar cheese
- ¼ cup Butter, cubed
- 1 cup Stuffing mix
- 1 teaspoon Mustard, grounded
- ¾ cup Walnuts, chopped
- Salt to taste

How to make it:

1. Clean the cauliflower, wash and dry and keep aside.
2. In a large bowl, put bouillon, sour cream, mustard and mix entirely.
3. Add cauliflower and mix the ingredients properly.
4. Transfer the mix to your keto Crockpot and set low cooking for about 2 hours.
5. Stir occasionally.
6. Once cooking is over, transfer it to a serving dish.
7. Take a large skillet and heat butter.
8. Add walnut and stuffing mix and toast it slightly and spread over the cooked food.
9. Serve hot.

Super-Food Frittata:

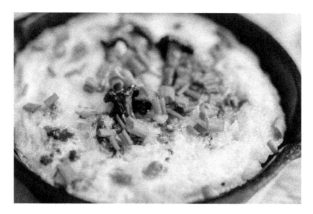

Serves: 6
Preparation Time: 15 minutes
Cooking Time: 3 hours
Macros per serving:
Calories: 180
Protein: 11.8 grams
Fat: 12.6 grams
Carbohydrates: 5.8 grams

What you'll need:

- 2 teaspoons olive oil
- 5 ounces fresh baby kale
- 6 ounces roasted red pepper, chopped finely
- ¼ cup chives, chopped
- 5 ounces feta cheese, crumbled
- 8 organic eggs, beaten
- ½ teaspoon spike seasoning
- Salt and freshly ground black pepper, to taste

How to make it:

1. Grease a Crockpot.
2. In a frying pan, heat oil over medium heat and sauté kale for about 3-4 minutes.
3. Transfer the kale into prepared Crockpot.
4. Add remaining ingredients apart from cheese and stir to mix. Sprinkle evenly with cheese.
5. Set the Crockpot on low and cook, covered, for about 2 hours 30 minutes - 3 hours.
6. Cut into 6 equal sized wedges and serve.

Eggplant Parmesan:

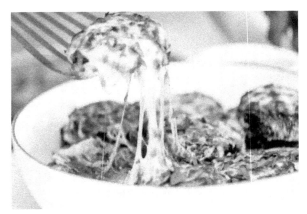

Serves: 2
Preparation Time: 40 minutes
Cooking Time: 4 hours
Macros per serving:
Calories: 159
Protein: 14 grams
Fat: 12 grams
Carbohydrates: 8 grams

What you'll need:

- 1 large eggplant, ½ -inch slices
- 1 egg, whisked
- 1 teaspoon Italian seasoning
- 1 cup marinara
- ¼ cup parmesan cheese, grated

How to make it:

1. Sprinkle each side of the eggplant with salt let stand for 30 minutes.
2. Spread the some of the marinara on the bottom of the Crockpot and season with salt and pepper, garlic powder and Italian seasoning.
3. Spread the eggplants on a single the Crockpot and pour over some of the marinara sauce. Repeat this for 2 to 3 layers.
4. Top with parmesan.
5. Cover and cook for 4 hours.

Cream of Mushroom Soup:

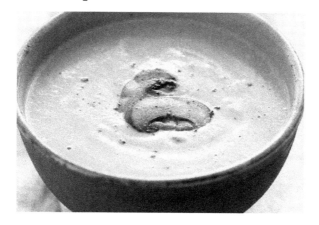

Serves: 4
Preparation Time: 6 minutes
Cooking Time: 3 hours
Macros per serving:
Calories: 229
Protein: 5 grams
Fat: 21 grams
Carbohydrates: 9 grams

What you'll need:

- 1 tablespoon olive oil
- ½ cup onion, diced
- 20 ounces mushrooms, sliced
- 2 cups chicken broth
- 1 cup heavy cream

How to make it:

1. In a skillet, heat the oil over medium flame and sauté the onions until translucent or slightly brown on the edges.
2. Transfer into Crockpot and add the mushrooms and chicken broth. Season with salt and pepper to taste.
3. Close the lid and cook on low for 6 hours or on high for 3 hours until the mushrooms are soft
4. Halfway before the cooking time ends, stir in the heavy cream.

Tasty Summer Squash:

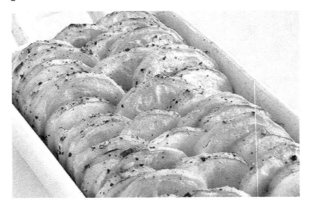

Serves: 4
Preparation Time: 10 minutes
Cooking Time: 2 hours
Macros per serving:
Calories: 98
Protein: 2.6 grams
Fat: 7.4 grams
Carbohydrates: 8.2 grams

What you'll need:

- 1 yellow summer squash, sliced
- 2 tablespoons water
- 2 medium zucchini, sliced
- 2 tablespoons olive oil
- Pepper
- Salt

How to make it:

1. Add all ingredients into the slow cooker and mix well.
2. Cover and cook on high for 2 hours.
3. Serve and enjoy.

Crockpot Green Bean Casserole:

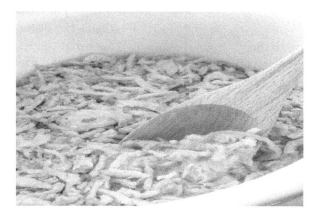

Serves: 8
Preparation Time: 15 minutes
Cooking Time: 4 hours
Macros per serving:
Calories: 300
Protein: 12 grams
Fat: 18 grams
Carbohydrates: 6 grams

What you'll need:

- 1 pound green bean, cooked
- 1/3 pound bacon, cooked & chopped

For Creamy Cheese Sauce:

- 3 ounces onion, finely minced
- 1 clove garlic, minced
- 4 tablespoons dry vermouth
- 1 tablespoon parsley, minced
- 1 teaspoon lemon zest
- 2 tablespoons bacon drippings
- 6 ounces cream cheese
- ¾ cup chicken broth
- 3 ounces cheddar cheese, grated
- 1 teaspoon Worcestershire sauce
- Salt to taste
- Pepper to taste

For topping:

- 1/3 cups Low carb bread crumbs
- 1/8 teaspoons Garlic, granulated
- Salt to taste
- 2 teaspoon Olive oil (use as required)

How to make it:

- In a small skillet cook beans and bacon by adding little water and after cooking drain and set aside.
- Medium heat a large skillet and add little bacon drippings.
- Add the minced onion and stir until becomes translucent.
- Then add garlic and continue stirring until it becomes soft.
- Slow down the heat and add parsley, wine, and lemon zest.
- Continue stirring for some time until the smell of the wine disappears.
- Now add the cream cheese and let it melt. Stir occasionally.
- Add chicken broth slowly and sauté occasionally.
- Add cheddar cheese, mustard, Worcestershire sauce, pepper, and salt and continue stirring.

- Transfer the mixture to the bowl of bacon and beans.
- Mix it properly.
- Transfer the entire mixture to the Crockpot and set for low cooking for about 4 hours.
- Make the topping. For that put the breadcrumbs into a small bowl. Add granulated garlic and salt as required along with olive oil as needed. Mix it properly and sprinkle on top of the dish.
- Check the dish occasionally and make sure that there is enough water for cooking. If it looks dry, you can some water or chicken broth.
- Serve hot.

Tummy Satisfying Casserole:

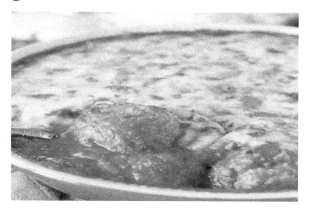

Serves: 8
Preparation Time: 20 minutes
Cooking Time: 7 hours
Macros per serving:
Calories: 415
Protein: 29.3 grams
Fat: 31.1 grams
Carbohydrates: 4.2 grams

What you'll need:

- ½ cup unsweetened almond milk
- 12 organic eggs
- ½ teaspoon dry mustard
- Salt and freshly ground black pepper, to taste
- 1 head cauliflower, shredded
- 1 small yellow onion, chopped
- 10-ounces cooked bacon, chopped
- 2 cups cheddar cheese, shredded

How to make it:

1. Grease a Crockpot.
2. In a bowl, add the milk eggs, mustard, salt, and black pepper and beat well.
3. In the bottom of prepared Crockpot, place about 1/3 of the cauliflower in an even layer, followed by 1/3 of the onion.
4. Sprinkle with salt and pepper.
5. Top with 1/3 of the bacon, followed by 1/3 of the cheese.
6. Repeat the layers twice and top with egg mixture.
7. Set the Crockpot on low and cook, covered, for about 5-7 hours.
8. Cut into 6 equal sized wedges and serve.

Garlic Ranch Mushrooms:

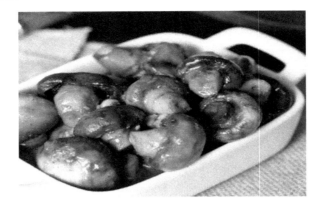

Serves: 2
Preparation Time: 10 minutes
Cooking Time: 2 hours
Macros per serving:
Calories: 97
Protein: 10 grams
Fat: 20 grams
Carbohydrates: 3 grams

What you'll need:

- 1 package of ranch dressing
- 4 package of whole mushrooms
- 1 cube butter, melted

How to make it:

1. Place 5 cloves of garlic at the bottom of the Crockpot and pour in the melted butter.
2. Add in the mushrooms and pour the dressing season with salt and pepper to taste.
3. Cover and cook on high for 2 hours.

Broccoli and Cheese Casserole:

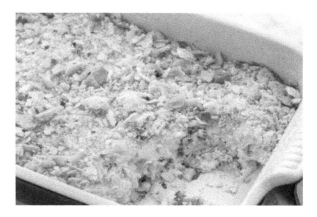

Serves: 4
Preparation Time: 5 minutes
Cooking Time: 4 hours
Macros per serving:
Calories: 78
Protein: 8.2 grams
Fat: 5.8 grams
Carbohydrates: 4 grams

What you'll need:

- ¾ cup almond flour
- 1 head of broccoli, cut into florets
- 2 large eggs, beaten
- Salt and pepper to taste
- ½ cup mozzarella cheese

How to make it:

1. Place the almond flour and broccoli in the Crockpot.
2. Stir in the eggs and season with salt and pepper to taste.
3. Sprinkle with mozzarella cheese.
4. Close the lid and cook on low for 4 hours or on high for 2 hours.

CONCLUSION:

Thank you for reading this book and having the patience to try the recipes.

I do hope that you gain as much enjoyment reading and experimenting with the meals as I have had writing these books.
If you would like to leave a comment, you can do it at the Order section->Digital order send and also buy paperback, in your Amazon account.

Stay safe and healthy!